The Healthy Girl's
GUIDE TO BREAST CANCER

Christine Egan

BALBOA.
PRESS

A DIVISION OF HAY HOUSE

Balboa Press books may be ordered through booksellers or by contacting:

Balboa Press
A Division of Hay House
1663 Liberty Drive
Bloomington, IN 47403
www.balboapress.com
1-(877) 407-4847

Because of the dynamic nature of the Internet, any web addresses or links contained in this book may have changed since publication and may no longer be valid. The views expressed in this work are solely those of the author and do not necessarily reflect the views of the publisher, and the publisher hereby disclaims any responsibility for them.

The author of this book does not dispense medical advice or prescribe the use of any technique as a form of treatment for physical, emotional, or medical problems without the advice of a physician, either directly or indirectly. The intent of the author is only to offer information of a general nature to help you in your quest for emotional and spiritual well-being. In the event you use any of the information in this book for yourself, which is your constitutional right, the author and the publisher assume no responsibility for your actions.

Any people depicted in stock imagery provided by Thinkstock are models, and such images are being used for illustrative purposes only.
Certain stock imagery © Thinkstock.

Printed in the United States of America.

ISBN: 978-1-4525-7459-2 (sc)
ISBN: 978-1-4525-7461-5 (hc)
ISBN: 978-1-4525-7460-8 (e)

Library of Congress Control Number: 2013908924

Balboa Press rev. date: 06/12/13

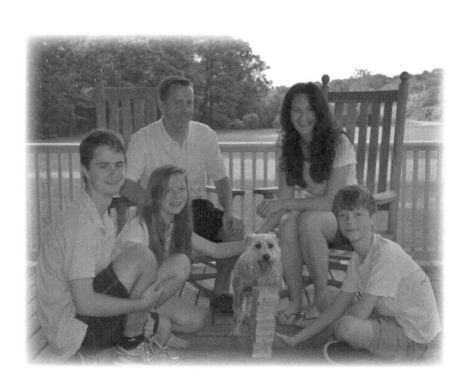

Dedication

This book is dedicated to my family: My husband Frank, my son Frank, my daughter Emily and my son Jack. Thank you for helping me realize the importance of the simple things in life.

Plain and simple…I love you.

Just because cancer has become ingrained in the public consciousness as a growing behemoth out of our control does not make it so. Shift the conversation, inspire change, and demand a life for yourself that is not driven by a fear of cancer or ruled by disease. There will always be others who want you to believe that such a thing is inevitable and that prevention is impossible, but those are the same people that feed on the hysteria and neglect the facts. We have the potential to quell cancer's onslaught by committing ourselves to a better understanding of what lifestyle behaviors are at the root of it, not just what options we are given on the operating table.

-Richard Linchitz, M.D. a 14-year cancer survivor and director of Linchitz Medical Wellness

Table of Contents

I'LL START OFF THANKING THE obvious people who helped me get this book into print. I thank my husband, Frank for not only being by my side during "that" time in our lives, but for encouraging me to start and finish this book project. My three kids: Frank, Emily and Jack for being such great sounding boards for ideas big and small. A huge debt of gratitude goes to my editor Suzanne Boothby; without your assistance this book would not have happened. You were constantly helping put my thoughts into words and reminding me that people want to hear what I have to say.

There were other people involved with the production of this book. My daughter, Emily I love the photo you took of me at the beach for the book cover. Kristine Scaglione, I thank you for taking my family photo and my author biography picture; I still don't know how you got all of us including the dog to look at the camera. A big thank you goes to my sister-in-law Janet Egan for getting the photos production ready.

Now I would like to thank everyone else that helped me along this cancer journey. A big fat hug goes to my tennis partner and friend Mary Lane. You gave me the needed strength during my early doctor appointments. To my friends who cared for me post-surgery: Tina Annibell for making my special detox tea. Margaret James for not only making me laugh during difficult times but for your bedside manner. And for the countless friends who stopped by with food for me and my family. For all the great staff at the various cancer treatment offices; I thank you for your compassion.

Two of my closest friends were touched by cancer. I thank Linda and Peggy for both helping me stay strong and for helping me figure out what other people need to hear when cancer touches their life.

Whether you cheered me on with Facebook posts or in person, I thank you for helping me get the word out about the importance of empowering yourself during a difficult and dark time.

Lastly, I thank my friends at my local Starbucks for letting me sit there for hours while I wrote this book! The Sayville morning crew is a bundle of positive energy.

You become what you believe, not what you wish.

—*Oprah Winfrey*

Introduction

I HAVE TO START BY letting you know this book isn't about cancer; it's about wellness. Tony Robbins asks, "What story are you telling yourself in your head?" The story I told myself was that I wasn't sick; I was healthy. That's right. I was a healthy person who just happened to have to deal with cancer. Cancer would not be my identity, and I would not be a walking billboard for it. I did want to be a billboard for health.

I always loved the idea of having a theme song. During my adventure with cancer, I had three songs that played non-stop in my head.

The first one I found while I was sitting in the chemotherapy treatment room. I was reclined in a dark brown leather chair surrounded by three young female nurses in hospital scrubs. My body was in a strangely semi-relaxed state, and I had a clear tube, twenty-four inches long, coming out of the upper right side of my chest. I could hear people talking to me, but it sounded more like mumbled background noise. The only words I could hear were the ones playing in my head. The sounds were from the eighties band the Talking Heads. I imagined hearing the following words repeated with a funky beat:

"You may ask yourself, well, how did I get here?
You may ask yourself, am I right, am I wrong?
You may say to yourself, my God, what have I done?"

I felt like I had written those words myself. They sum up my cancer experience in three little lines.

I didn't remember the name of that song until I started to write this book. I think the title is very appropriate for me: "Once In a Lifetime." I still cling to the thought that this cancer adventure happened once in my lifetime.

You'll hear more about the other songs as we go. Stay tuned.

How I Came to Write This Book

The idea of writing a book started out as a joke. Whenever I met new doctors or their staff, I would tell them to be nice to me because I was writing a book and wouldn't want them portrayed poorly. It was a fun way to break the ice with doctors' offices, and it helped the staff remember me. The other silly line I used often was "Whoever sees my naked breast has to get in a picture with me." If there was a doctor or staff member who was lucky enough to see my breast, they were lucky enough to get in a picture with me. It was fun when I walked into an office and people said, with a smile on their face, "Oh yeah, we heard about you."

The book began as a way to help me heal. I didn't want years to go by and let regret creep in. I wanted a place to capture my feelings about my time with cancer. My goal was to get my story down on paper while the thoughts were still fresh in my head.

As I wrote, the universe kept encouraging me to move forward with my book. I would write in the morning, and then I would run into someone later that day who reinforced something I had just been writing about. I would hear stories about friends struggling to find their way in the health care system. People who didn't know I had cancer would comment on how great my skin and hair looked. Friends would ask me details about radiation. Someone actually asked me if my breast was black and charred from it. Right then, I heard the universe confirming that it was important for me to write a book. I could tell people about my experience and give them details about my treatment. I wanted to demystify breast cancer. With information comes power, and I want others to be powerful if this should happen to them, their family member, or their friend.

I also wanted to write this book because I felt like a mountain climber who had reached my summit. I now have this incredible view that I want to share. There are still many climbers down below, and not every climber takes the same way up.

Let's get clear about a few things. I am not a doctor or a nurse, nor have I studied cancer for years. Thank goodness! I am new to cancer. As I write this, it has been in my life for only a little more than a year. Before my diagnosis, I knew people who had cancer, but it did not affect my life as profoundly until I got my own news. I quickly took it upon myself to become chief medical researcher (of cancer material), a great interviewer (of doctors), and a healthy chef (for myself and my family). I took responsibility for my body and my treatment. I never left any decision to be made solely by a medical practitioner. I did research, asked questions, said no, said yes, and when I needed to, kept my head down to get through what was needed to get well.

My intention is simple: I want to retell my story and shed some light on how I handled a difficult situation with a healthy twist. I want to let you know how I stayed positive, strong, and somewhat sane during the cancer circus. During my one-year unthinkable journey of cancer, I have navigated the health care system, made life-changing decisions, and all the while maintained a positive outlook on life. Some things helped me along the way, and I decided they were too important not to share with you.

So how did a healthy, unsuspecting mother and wife get breast cancer at forty-two?

Sometimes I catch myself looking at visibly unhealthy people and think, *I'm the one with cancer? How is that possible?! I'm the person who eats healthier than most, exercises, avoids prescription drugs, and meditates. Yet I'm the one with cancer.*

I try not to dwell on the how or why, because the truth is I will never know why I got it and the woman next to me didn't. The question interests me, though, because if I could figure out what I did, then it seems like I could figure out what to do so it never returns. Was it the water? The food? The stress? The thyroid troubles? The environment? The genes? The list goes on and on. But I will never know the exact cause. All I know is that I thought I was doing everything right.

So this book isn't about the why or the how of cancer, but about my journey as a healthy person navigating the health care system, staying positive, and remaining healthy throughout.

This book will inform you about some alternative cancer treatments that I researched and participated in. I'm not out to persuade you that one treatment is better than another, but I will tell you what worked for me. I want you to feel empowered to choose what is right for you. I want you to own your body and take charge of it, because only you can take charge of your health. As you read, you will see that I did not follow conventional treatments. I armed myself with knowledge and power. And you can do that too!

Unfortunately, everyone these days has a connection to cancer. Every nineteen seconds someone in the world gets a breast cancer diagnosis, according to the Institute for Health Metrics and Evaluation, University of Washington. These days you would be hard-pressed to find someone who hasn't been through it themselves or doesn't know someone—a family member or friend—who has. My hope is that with more awareness we can all improve our well-being. I hope my story can serve as a guide to others who are struggling with their own news.

Before cancer my life was moving along quite merrily. I lived in an upscale neighborhood, just steps from the Great South Bay on Long Island. I lived in a beautiful three-story house, surrounded by a garden with an in-ground pool and a hot tub. My days consisted of running kids to dance, karate, and sailing—all while putting good, healthy meals together. I truly appreciated my life. My husband, Frank, and I taught Pre-Cana (marriage preparation class for the Catholic Church) yearly, which we did selfishly because it made us fall in love all over again.

I worked part time in Frank's orthodontic office doing the behind-the-scenes work, including marketing and special projects. I really enjoyed my time at the office, because I knew that it made Frank's life a little easier. The office was doing really well and ran mostly on autopilot at this point.

The homeschooling of our three kids was getting much easier. The days of angst about whether or not we were doing the right thing by homeschooling the kids had disappeared. They had become such self-starters that the non-school time was now filled with reading, online classes, and fun projects. The three kids were close and usually a joy to be around. I loved having them home and being on our own schedule. Our family loved having downtime together without the constraints of a school schedule. The kids are very close with both sets of grandparents, and I know that if they were in regular school, they would not enjoy such a strong bond.

I had just finished a yearlong program at the Institute for Integrative Nutrition to become a certified health coach. The year at school reminded me how much fun it was to follow my passion about healthy food. I traveled to New York City twice a month for my classes and loved every second of it! I loved meeting new people who were passionate about food. Every month I would learn about different dietary theories and the effects on the body. Classes were held in a huge theater, and the school hosted some of the premier doctors, authors, and researchers I had watched for the previous twenty years. That meant every class was like attending a concert with my favorite rock stars. It really inspired me to take my healthy eating to a new level. The program also included plenty of self-discovery. I was forced to think about what it took to make me happy and where I see myself in the future.

The school's founder, Joshua Rosenthal, says, "Someone can eat broccoli all day long and still be unhealthy." One of his big philosophies is that the foods you eat are secondary to all other things that feed you. Your family, career, exercise, and spirituality all play a role in creating a healthy, balanced individual. Joshua says, "We are fed not by food, but by the energy in our lives." This theory opened my eyes to see the many pieces of the health puzzle. I took it with me while I navigated my cancer adventure, knowing not one type of healthy food was going to heal me or one type of cancer treatment was going to cure me. It was going to take a series of healthy habits to put me back into balance.

The school trained me to have an open mind and explore more options for healing. I can't imagine my cancer journey without the tools of understanding my mind, body, and soul on a deeper level. My school also taught me how to "fit out." Instead of trying to be like everyone else, you can actually work to be just as you are—speak up for what you want and not be afraid to stand out from the crowd. We are all conditioned to fit in, but once you start fitting out, you start to understand the power of your own beat. This idea served me well in cancer treatment. I had the courage to listen to my own wisdom and not follow all of the "rules."

Although many people reach out, only you alone can take the cancer journey. Yes, people were there for me during surgeries, treatments, and decisions, but I was the one who had to go ahead and endure them. I was the one who thought about cancer 24/7 for the first few months. I'm not saying others around me weren't affected. I'm just saying it's something that you do alone. But I hope in sharing my story, I can become someone who supports you during this time. If I can do it, you can too.

Chapter 1

My Journey from Grilled Cheese to Grilled Veggies

WELL, I WASN'T ALWAYS THE healthy woman I am today. I grew up on Long Island eating food from packages (sorry, Mom!). Although my mother tried to encourage me to eat vegetables, I never would. My cousins still, to this day, love reminding me of the time my aunt made me eat canned string beans with dinner and I proceeded to throw them up hours later on the floor of the dining room.

Growing up, my favorite foods included anything sweet. I will confess that many a breakfast consisted of a wrapped chocolate cake: think Hostess, Drake, or Entenmann's. There wasn't a Yodel or Yankee Doodles cupcake that I would refuse. Our family dinners consisted of some kind of meat and a potato, and I was always the last to finish. I would come up with creative ways to hide my uneaten food: underneath the rim of my plate, in my napkin, or—my favorite—in the bottom of my milk cup. Later, when I was off at college, I wasn't much better. I think I ate grilled cheese for lunch and dinner for most of my college years. My friends back then called me the Dairy Queen. My love of sweets and ice cream didn't change as I got older.

After college, I landed a job with the same advertising agency that I had interned with in New York. The position I was offered was in Detroit, Michigan. I was happy to get a job after graduation, and the idea of moving to another big city really appealed to me. My life became filled with work. I loved my job, I loved the people I was surrounded with, I loved being in another big city, and I was happy with my life. I positioned myself as a very hard worker, putting in six days a week and making myself available at all hours. I had great movie role models of working women back then. Remember Melanie Griffith in *Working Girl* and Holly Hunter in *Broadcast News*? These two women made it okay to be powerful and hardworking. I so wanted to be them! I had visions of climbing the corporate ladder and making a lifelong career for myself in advertising.

Back then, my diet still wasn't great. Breakfast, if any, was usually coffee and a pastry. Lunch was a take-out sandwich from a deli. Dinner probably consisted of the free hors d'oeuvres from the local bar while out with coworkers. It took me several months of living on my own to understand that food could affect the way I felt. My health food epiphany came when I shared a house with a girl from Italy who never ate anything from a box. Daniela made cake from scratch. I thought cake from scratch meant opening a box of Duncan Hines. I'm not kidding! I never had a "homemade" cake that wasn't from a box. Daniela opened my eyes to real foods: fruits and vegetables. I tasted fresh vegetables, not from a can or the freezer. I remember having fresh string beans with shallots and olive oil and loving them (not throwing them up)! I recall details of eating my first roasted beet—that sweet, earthy flavor was something I never would have enjoyed years earlier. Daniela even started a little garden in the backyard where she grew her own tomatoes. I can still see her making her homemade tomato sauce at the kitchen stove. I slowly started cooking my own meals, which included fresh vegetables.

Once I opened my eyes to eating better, I started going to the local health food store with guidance from a coworker, Linda. I can recall the strange smells that filled the store. It was like a supermarket, but I didn't recognize the items on the shelves. The people who filled the store were happy, and patrons lingered in the small café. I sampled some of their prepared foods'some I liked, but some had strange textures or smells that I couldn't get past. It was a whole new environment. I tried different cereals like oatmeal rather than a top-selling box type. I started eating more fruits and vegetables and gradually adding healthy foods to my life.

My health transformation didn't happen overnight; it was a process. Part of my job was to visit McDonald's restaurants and eat their food. It was my job to get people to buy McDonald's food. Back then, I didn't have a problem with that; nowadays, I would.

During the next ten years, I paid more attention to health. I did a lot of experimenting with different foods and ways of eating. I ate meat, and then I gave it up for a while; then I started eating it again. I bought a juicer. I learned where all the health food stores were in my neighborhood. As I made healthier food choices and felt better in my body, I noticed other parts of my life were not working so well. I was working for a company I didn't like. I was in a relationship I wasn't happy in. Something had to change.

I quit my job after seven years, left a long-term relationship, and moved back to Long Island. I left the advertising world, and went back to school and became a licensed massage therapist. I reconnected with my high school boyfriend. He didn't know it, but he had stayed on my mind all those years. Frank was just about to finish his ten years of schooling. He was in his last semester of his orthodontic residency. It seemed that both of us had finally made room in our lives for each other. We got married, bought a house and an orthodontic office, and settled down to have a baby, all within two years. Life was good, and I was happy. I seemed to be living the life I was meant to have.

Fast-forward to my first pregnancy. I remember reading and watching TV shows about childbirth, thinking I wanted to do it differently. Okay, let's be honest here. I have a real phobia about needles. I have always been fearful of IVs in my arm or hand as well as having to give blood. I was so afraid of getting the IV put into my arm for the birth of my child that I thought, *if I can deliver this baby naturally, I won't need the IV.* I found a doctor's office that also had a midwife on staff. I made all my appointments with the midwife. My thought process was *this is a naturally occurring event, so why add interventions unless necessary?* I researched natural childbirth, took classes, and prepared fully for the experience. I was ready!

I successfully gave birth to my son, Frank, without any medical interventions: no IV, no spinal medication, no vaginal cutting, no stitches, no nothing! Frank was born at midnight, and we left the next morning. It was great! I felt fantastic.

Although I had quit my career in advertising, I didn't see myself in the role of a mother, either. I loved being a mother, but I really grappled with being a stay-at-home mom. I started working in my husband's orthodontic office at the front desk as a way to get out of the house and help him at the same time.

Life back then was a blur, and two years later, I was pregnant again. Since the first birth had gone so well (and was so uneventful), we decided to have our next child at home. Yes, you read that right ... at home! Besides finding the right home-birthing midwife, Frank and I took classes and became certified childbirth educators. With the help of a home-birth midwife, we prepared to have this child right in our second-story bedroom.

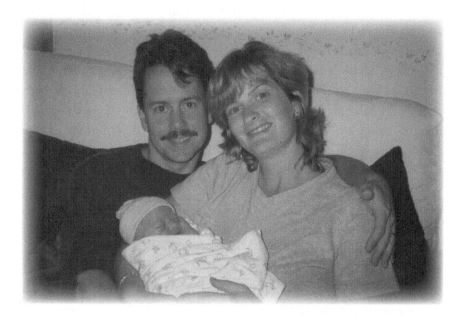

This picture was taken the day Emily was born at home.

The pregnancy went well. Again, I was ready to trust my body to do what it needed to do. I went into labor on Wednesday night before dinnertime. I hung out in the pool for a few hours while one-year-old Frank played near me in the shallow end. We put him to bed around eight, and I labored through the night. The midwife came over around six thirty in the morning, and Emily was born at 7:40 a.m., right on our bedroom floor. It was an incredible experience. Again, I was on top of the world, fully appreciating what my body was capable of doing. The highlight of the day was getting up to make a cake (from scratch) to celebrate Emily's true birthday. I felt invincible!

I intended to have another home birth for my third and final baby, but that didn't happen. Toward the end of my pregnancy, around thirty-eight weeks, I realized the baby wasn't moving as much as he had been. All the "natural" ideas went out the window, and medical intervention stepped in. Jack was born via C-section at the hospital and then put into the neonatal intensive care unit because he was so small at just under four pounds. It was a very stressful time for us as a family, wondering whether Jack was mentally and physically okay. He is fine now, but it was scary while it was all happening. Besides the stress of a newborn, I needed to let my body heal from the trauma of an emergency C-section.

I share those birthing stories with you so you can understand more about how we (my husband, Frank, and I) have dealt with various situations. We tend to view things a little differently from most people. We like to read and research different ways to treat things many people think are "normal." Yet we are not blind to when true medical intervention is needed. *We didn't just do what society expected us to do;* we did what was right for us. This approach would serve us well ten years later, as you will see.

Chapter 2

How Did the Healthiest Girl in the Room Get Cancer?

I HAVE ALWAYS BEEN ONE of those organized people, making my yearly ob-gyn visit right around my birthday in November. Well, I went to see my doctor; he did a breast exam, and it was all clear. He gave me a prescription for my mammogram, yet something inside me asked him for a script for an ultrasound as well. I had already had my baseline mammogram done less than five years before. I remember the technician saying I had dense breasts; I assumed most people did. I had to go back for a separate appointment for the ultrasound the first time around. I didn't understand that dense, heavy breasts needed an ultrasound because the mammogram does not show as much as the ultrasound.

I wanted to make things simpler this time around. My doctor gave me the prescriptions for both the mammogram and ultrasound so I could do both in the same appointment. I remember thinking I would make the appointment after the holidays.

About four weeks later, I was lying on the couch with my hand under my head, watching a movie, when my twenty-five-pound dog Zoe walked on top of me and started pawing at my left breast. I remember thinking it was strange. What the heck was Zoe doing? It was one of those moments that I had an intuitive feeling I was supposed to pay attention to. For some reason I trusted my gut and started to massage my left breast for a quick second.

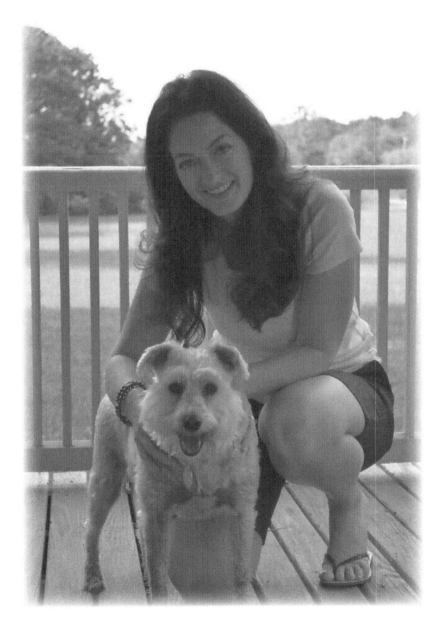

Our schnoodle Zoe.

That's when I felt the lump. It was on the upper left part of my breast. It felt like a BB bullet—a small, round, superficial mass. I had felt a mass like this before when I was breast-feeding and it had turned out to be a clogged milk duct. I remember thinking it was odd to be feeling a clogged milk duct at that point since it had been nearly ten years since I had last breast-fed. I reassured myself that it must be muscle I was feeling since I had recently increased my free weights at kickboxing.

I put the lump out of my mind, kind of. I didn't want to deal with it until after the holidays. But its presence stayed with me. I would feel it in the shower. It was still there. I would feel it before I went to bed. It was still there. I wasn't ready to make the time to go to the doctor with the holidays approaching, but there was a nagging deep down in my gut that I could not ignore.

I made the appointment with the breast center for my mammography and ultrasound at the beginning of January. The day of my appointment I drove alone and was a total wreck. I remember walking into the mammogram room and feeling really sick to my stomach and lightheaded. I never said a word to the technician about the lump. I figured if it *was* something, they would find it. I recall the squeezing of the mammography machine for both breasts and thinking, *Thank God that's over*. The films were then brought back to the radiologist down the hall to be read. I sat in the mammography room in a chair in the corner almost hyperventilating. I tried to use my deep abdominal yoga breath to calm down, as my heart was racing and my armpits were sweating. I was relieved I was in the hospital gown, because my armpits drenched it.

The technician walked back into the room and said I was all clear. Wow—it really was nothing. I was feeling a sense of relief. The medical technician escorted me down the hall to a different room for the ultrasound test. I was still nervous, but felt like the appointment was almost over and that my "mass" was nothing.

The ultrasound room was very different from the mammogram room. There was no big machine or bright lights, and it had an examining table to lie down on. The computer in the corner played acoustic-type music. The ultrasound technician and I made small talk about reality TV shows and our kids while she slathered my breast in K-Y jelly to help the ultrasound wand glide over my breast. Then it happened. She found it.

The tech turned to me and said, "There is a lump here. Are you aware of it?"

I confessed that I was aware of it. She finished with the ultrasound wand on my left breast. Then she moved on to the right breast. When she was finished, she said she needed to get the radiologist to look at the ultrasound report. I remember waiting on the exam table, trying to wipe K-Y jelly from my breasts, and again attempting to use that calming yoga breathing to ease my nerves.

The doctor came back within five minutes with a look of seriousness. He said he did not like the way the mass looked and that I needed to get a core needle biopsy.

"Okay, when can I do it?" I asked.

"ASAP," he replied in an urgent tone.

I had never met this doctor before, but I could tell he was saying this lump was serious. I knew deep down that ASAP wasn't good. I got dressed, and the ultrasound technician walked me to the front desk. She helped me make the appointment for Wednesday (it was Monday). I knew from the technician and the radiologist that this was serious.

I went home not making a big deal of it. I did not research breast lumps on the computer, because I knew that I could not handle even thinking about "what if." I told myself I was healthy, this was just a scare, and everything would be fine.

I went back to the breast center by myself two days later for the core needle biopsy, not knowing what I was getting myself into. If I had taken the time to dissect the word, I might have been more prepared. A *needle* was involved, and *biopsy* meant they were taking a sample of the mass. It never occurred to me what was about to happen.

A different technician took me back to the ultrasound room and explained that I needed to get undressed with the gown open in the front. She told me to lie down on the table and she would be back soon. Before the technician left, I explained to her how nervous I was and that I needed her to help me through this.

"No problem," she said. "I will be by your side while the doctor does the procedure."

The technician and doctor came in and redid the ultrasound first, locating the mass. Once that was done, a needle was inserted into my breast to numb it. I felt the pinching, but the pain was manageable. The next needle was the one that literally went into the mass and took out a small tissue sample to be tested for cancer. Now the tears were streaming down my face in fear, not in pain. Once the sample was removed, a metal piece—a.k.a. "marker"—was inserted into my breast, so that the mass could be found easily again. The pain was not intense, just uncomfortable. I couldn't wrap my head around this metal piece being left in me—somehow that didn't seem right. Once the doctor was finished with the biopsy portion, I needed another mammogram to indicate the location of the "marker" that was left behind. Then the waiting game began.

I don't even remember the time between the biopsy and the results. I think cancer was just the furthest thing from my mind. I didn't think "it" could happen to me.

A week later I received a call from my ob/gyn. Coincidentally, his wife had also had breast cancer a few years earlier.

"I hate to tell you this, but you have breast cancer," he said. "You are going to be fine—it's the early stage—but you need to make some calls."

I remember taking the call in the living room, but when he started talking to me, I walked into the basement so I could be alone. I let the tears come as I wrote down information, because I hadn't thought about the next steps. I had never let myself think of the "what-ifs." It was one of those times when my mind was a blank and my body was still. I listened to my doctor talk about the biopsy results, but didn't understand any of it. I just took notes. I asked him about referrals to doctors, and he rattled off the names of a couple of breast surgeons to call.

I hung up the phone and walked upstairs to my husband and kids. I turned at the top of the stairs. Frank looked at me and knew something was wrong, but couldn't in a million years figure out what. Then I blurted out, "I have cancer."

He hugged me and we cried together. I told the kids right then and there too. I think the only one who understood the magnitude of it all was my fourteen-year-old son, Frank.

He turned to me and said, "God has a plan; let's see what it is."

I wasn't quite sure how to take my son's wisdom. I remember feeling relieved and uneasy at the same time.

I immediately sprang into action, making calls, crying to receptionists on the phone, and gathering information about what the heck I was supposed to do next. I made appointments with four different breast surgeons. Once the action part was complete, I was left with the feelings and so many questions.

I am a young, healthy mother and wife. How could this happen to my family and me?

How could my body go against me?

The same body that created three beautiful children, that ran a half marathon just a few months ago, eats mostly organic foods

How could this happen? And to my breast? I love my breasts!

Chapter 3

Okay, I Have Breast Cancer: Now What?

WHEN THE DEVASTATING WORDS *You have Cancer* were spoken to me, I thought I would do anything to keep myself alive for my family. I couldn't even think about not being there for my three young children or my husband of fourteen years.

Cancer is a scary word. I was so scared of cancer that I was ready to follow blindly into mainstream cancer treatment and do what I needed to do to stay alive. I looked to doctors to provide the answers to my problem. But I also tried to remember that these doctors treat many, many, many cancer patients on a daily basis. And guess what? I was not a typical cancer patient! I could not answer yes to any one of the "precancer" questions I was asked: I ate the right foods, I exercised, I had started menstruating at the "right" age, I breast-fed my kids, I was not on birth control pills, and I didn't smoke or do recreational drugs.

It was difficult not to just let the medical establishment lead me in the direction they wanted me to go. I know I've read that when people go into a doctor's office, they revert to childlike behavior. I can attest to that. I am a highly intelligent woman who doesn't go into things blindly, and I found it difficult to navigate the medical community by myself.

The next step was to choose a breast surgeon and deal with all the doctors and medical experts. I was already familiar with best-selling author Kris Carr and her book, *Crazy, Sexy, Cancer.* I remember reading that when she interviewed various doctors, she acted like the CEO of her body. I took this attitude as well. I too wanted to put together a Board of

Directors—a team of doctors, friends, and family who listened to me and treated me with dignity and respect.

As the CEO of my body, I decided it was my responsibility to figure out which option was best for me. It was my job to do what was best for my body. Period. I came to realize that no one in the medical community had all the right answers or a magic cure. No doctor—or even nondoctor, for that matter—can tell you what to do. The doctors serve as the reference guides. Each one has a piece of the information, but it is up to you to gather what you need from each one and decide which course of action is best for you.

I created my own cancer timetable as well. I was not in a life-threatening situation, so I took my time assembling the best Board of Directors to help me beat cancer. I was out to find the right team of doctors and the best treatment, and create a timetable that worked for me. I managed my own health care. By taking control of my situation and researching different cancer treatments, I felt informed and empowered.

Being your own CEO comes with a lot of responsibility. If you feel like you are not up to the task, then ask someone you trust to help you. Having a friend or family member help you make decisions can be helpful. But it is important for you and them to understand that each decision is ultimately yours.

Let the Interview Process Begin

The next stop on my cancer adventure was to start interviewing breast surgeons. My gynecologist gave me a few different names. I started calling. It was extremely difficult to make that first call. What was I supposed to say? I really had no idea what to say or ask for.

"Hi, I have cancer. I need help."

How awkward, right? I did not want to share this horrible intimate detail of my life with the receptionist on the other end of the line. But somehow I found what worked for me.

I would say something like, "Yes, I need to see the surgeon. I was just diagnosed with breast cancer."

Sometimes I would cry as they went through the next set of questions, sometimes I wouldn't. It just seemed unthinkable that I would be saying

I had cancer out loud. Most of the calls were the same: they gathered insurance information and personal information, and always ended with a list of "requirements" that doctor needed: films, a CD version—some even needed the tissue sample from the biopsy.

I managed to line up appointments with four different breast surgeons. My friend Mary, who is a nurse practitioner, came with me for most of the early appointments. You might be wondering why Frank didn't come with me. It was logistical. I didn't want Frank to take off from work while I interviewed doctors. I wanted to save him for when I really needed him. Mary was my note taker, my second set of ears, and someone whose opinion I counted on to help me decide which doctor was going to get the job of cutting cancer out of me.

So off we went to doctor number one. The office was about thirty minutes from my house and within a large medical building. The surgeon's small office was on the third floor. He was a single practitioner and an older man in his midsixties. Mary and I sat in the waiting room while I filled out paperwork. The tedious process of paperwork gets old real fast. After about fifteen minutes of filing out papers, and showing my insurance card and picture id we were called from the waiting area. I remember that I was not overly nervous, scared, and unsure, but I knew I was just on a fact-finding mission. I was determined to interview the right people to help make up that "Board of Directors," and that's how I viewed this appointment—purely as an interview.

We were led directly into an exam room. The nurse told me to get undressed and put on the paper gown. The doctor came in and introduced himself. He was nice enough, and had been treating breast cancer patients for thirty-plus years. He reviewed my biopsy report and ultrasound. He then proceeded to do a quick physical exam of my left breast. He explained that he would remove the cancer with a lumpectomy, which meant an incision in my left breast to remove the cancer mass.

I didn't like something about his bedside manner. He was very quick and to the point. He didn't describe the surgery to me in detail, as if I wouldn't understand. He acted as if his ways were the only option open to me, but I knew I was interviewing him and looking to make a real connection with someone with whom I would potentially be spending years. Neither Mary nor I liked him. He wasn't the one for me.

I compare interviewing cancer doctors to sorority pledging back in college. When I interviewed sororities in the mid-80s, all the different sorority houses were nice, but there was only one that made me feel like it was where I belonged.

Mary and I sat in my car reviewing the appointment when it occurred to her that she should call an oncologist she knew from her work at the hospital. He was young and at top of his game with a wait list several months out. Yet I was not thrilled by the idea of seeing an oncologist. Oncology equaled cancer. Visiting the breast surgeon's office was one thing, but visiting an oncologist's office was something totally different. In my mind, the breast surgeon did not equal cancer. It was a simple procedure, and I was hoping I wouldn't need the other treatment options.

I really thought I could escape a visit to the oncologist or at least postpone it for as long as possible. But I had to take advantage of any connections I had. As Mary called Dr. V's cell phone, I felt sick to my stomach. I didn't want to fully face the reality of cancer just yet, and at the oncologist's office, cancer would be front and center. She explained to him my diagnosis, and the next thing I knew, I had an appointment at the oncologist's office first thing the next morning.

Although I didn't like having it as my second doctor's visit, I was grateful to Mary. I knew she'd be there with me. I knew her personal connection to him would make for a less stressful visit.

I met Mary in the parking lot of the office at eight in the morning the next day. I was numb. I couldn't believe that cancer was going to be thrown in my face so fast. The office was like a mini hospital. I walked in and felt immediately confused. With about ten different sliding glass windows all filled with various instructions, I wasn't even sure where to sign in. I looked for the doctor's name and eventually found the right spot to hand in the paperwork that had been e-mailed to me the night before.

Mary and I sat in the empty waiting room, which could easily seat one hundred patients or more. She attempted to make small talk with me as we settled in. Luckily, they called my name within ten minutes. We were escorted to a mini laboratory filled with noisy blood-spinning machines, racks of empty and full blood vials, large computer screens full of patient information, a scale, and several of those chairs that have extended armrests for taking blood. I was told to sit at the chair with the arm extended. My pulse was racing, because I was afraid the next step was to have my blood drawn, but instead my finger got pricked for a baseline blood test. Then I got weighed and directed to an examining room. After a few minutes, Matt, a young medical assistant in his late twenties, entered the room to gather more of my medical information and to collect blood. Now, you know how I hate the blood part. So not only was I now at as an oncologist's office, but I also had to give blood!

I made small talk with Matt and found out he was expecting his first child in a few months. He told me he was used to dealing with much more difficult veins to access and that mine were easy to find. He took my blood with ease. With all that blood behind me, I was ready for the next step—to see the oncologist. Dr. V came into the room, and I was a little thrown when I saw he was my age, dressed in regular clothes, and cute. He hugged Mary and introduced himself to me with a hug and told me I was going to be fine. This meeting was the best I could have hoped for at this stage of my treatment.

He reviewed my biopsy report, performed a quick physical exam to feel the breast lump, and palpated my neck and armpits, looking for enlarged lymph nodes. Then he rattled off a bunch of tests he wanted me to have. None of them meant anything to me because I hadn't done any research on cancer treatments yet. Mary sat in the chair feverishly taking notes.

My appointment lasted more than sixty minutes. Dr. V was very generous with his time, allowing me to ask questions without feeling rushed. He told me to come back six weeks after my surgery and we would figure out the next steps for cancer treatments. He doubted that I would need the dreaded chemotherapy, based on the size of the cancerous mass and my excellent health. He said my cancer was detected early and he doubted that it had spread to other parts of my body. He felt confident that radiation and hormone therapy were the only treatments I would need besides the lumpectomy. Before I left, he gave me the name of a breast surgeon he thought would be a perfect fit for me. He even had someone in his office call over to her office to ensure I was seen that day.

Mary and I sat in my car, so happy that Dr. V didn't think I would need chemotherapy. We just sat there crying with joy. For the first time in a week I thought, *Okay, I can do this. I can handle the surgery and radiation.*

Next, I was off to doctor number three. This was the breast surgeon Dr. V had recommended. The office squeezed me in as the last appointment that day. Unfortunately, Mary could not come with me and Frank was at work, so I went alone. I filled out the same paperwork yet again. I remember crying when I handed in the stack of papers, because at this point I was exhausted after the oncologist visit that morning and having to do this appointment on my own. Joan, the receptionist, calmed me down by telling me I was in good hands and just showed me some much-needed sympathy.

Doctor number three came into the room and immediately put me at ease because she wanted to talk to me as a person, not just look at my breast. Dr. McCloy asked me about my cancer story. I told her about my dog Zoe, and she was very interested in my story. I proceeded to cry and tell her how scared I was about the diagnosis. Dr. McCloy listened and sympathized with me. She explained that she would do a lumpectomy and based on her findings would determine my next course of treatment. I knew this was the doctor for me, but I wanted to stay true to myself and interview the rest of the doctors I had scheduled.

Doctor number four was with a large, well-known hospital. It took much longer to get an appointment with her. I had to wait four weeks to get an appointment. This surgeon also wanted tissue samples of my biopsy, so it took time to get that shipped from the lab. With Mary by my side again, we waited for more than an hour in this posh waiting room. We chitchatted, made ourselves tea, and entertained ourselves with their library. This facility was also like a hospital setting, only with the attempt to be fancy. Nice wing-backed chairs, fish tanks, and large windows letting the outside light in really had an effect. When we finally got in to see the doctor, we were escorted up the elevator to the second floor and then down a long dark hallway. The visit was similar to the other two surgeon visits. First came the stack of paperwork, and then the physical exam, followed by the sit-down with the doctor. The breast surgeon led us to her private office and explained that she too recommended a lumpectomy. I liked this doctor but didn't like the large-scale facility. I really felt like I was just one of many cancer patients seen in a day. Also this facility treated only cancer patients, and I didn't want to be surrounded by so much cancer.

I had another interview scheduled in New York City with another surgeon, but by this time I had already decided which doctor I wanted. It was Dr. Colleen McCloy. I later found out she was close to my age and the mother of three children close in age to my three. I had this feeling that she would take care of me because I could easily have been one of her friends. It felt good as CEO of my body to be able to trust my decision about my surgeon.

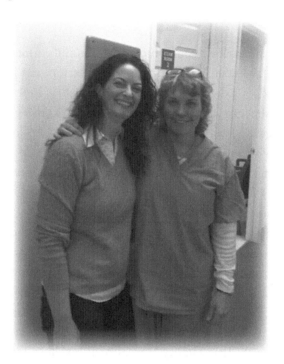

Me and my surgeon, Dr.Colleen McCloy.

I want to add something important here. I explained already how I listened to my gut when Jack wasn't moving inside of me, and again when Zoe was scratching at my breast. My gut was telling me something again. It was telling me that my cancer was something that would not take over my life. My gut was telling me this was not going to define me and that I would be healthy again soon. I remember being alone with my thoughts and knowing deep down that I was going to be okay. I would deal with this cancer and that would be it. I remember trying to cling to this feeling because I could see that there was a long road ahead of me, and I didn't want to get lost in this cancer mentality.

I was already starting to see that it was a struggle to remember that I was strong and healthy. With doctor visits, blood work, and nonstop medical paperwork, I was feeling a pull to jump down the despair hole. A book title popped into my mind—*When You Are Engulfed in Flames* by David Sedaris. Do you know the book? He tells the story of when he was in Paris and the back of his hotel door gave directions for what to do when you are on fire. The joke is that it's too late at that point, right? Who is going to read a sign once they are on fire? I knew I had cancer, but my body felt fine. I knew my journey would be mind over matter. I just had to remember not to get engulfed in the flames.

THINGS THAT HELPED ME DEAL WITH DOCTORS AND STAFF:

1. I made a conscious effort to be super nice to the staff. I let them know I was nervous and scared. I would start by striking up a conversation with them. I would ask the staff about their job or their family. They were usually very happy to talk. One of the staff members I first met at my oncologist's office was having a baby in a few months. I asked him questions about the baby preparations. This relaxed me when he took my blood pressure and blood work. People who work in cancer offices want to help and be friendly—I just needed to give them a reason to be. This chitchat usually helped me relax and helped people remember me each time I came in. I was no longer a faceless cancer patient.

2. I always had either my spouse or a friend with me. They would take notes while the doctor was examining me. Doctors will just talk and spout off information. It's important to get it all down. I knew that no matter how much I wanted to pay attention to what the doctor was saying, it was difficult to follow along because I recognized my emotional state was not always good when I went in for appointments. Sometimes I was nervous and scared; sometimes I would be distracted or unnerved from seeing other cancer patients around the office. The notes would help me remember everything that happened in that visit.

3. *I brought note cards with my questions to appointments.* Sometimes I got to the appointment knowing I wanted to ask XYZ, but the doctor would talk about something else, and I'd never get around to asking my questions. Having note cards with my questions ready to go helped me remember what I wanted to discuss.

4. *I would reread and then rewrite all my notes after each appointment.* This step might sound like overkill, but I wanted to make sure I understood all the scribbled notes from each appointment. I would review the notes while sitting in the car after the appointment to make sure I understood them and could ask questions as needed next time.

5. *Doctors are usually trained in one specific area or specialty.* The surgeon usually sees all breasts; the oncologist sees only cancer; the radiation oncologist deals only with the radiation portion of your treatment. They are surrounded only by what they are trained in—even the alternative doctors. It was important for me to remember that when I asked a question outside of the realm of their specialty, I understood where their information was coming from. It was my job to connect the dots later and ultimately oversee my treatment.

6. *Doctors are used to seeing many patients in a day.* I wanted to find a doctor who did not make me feel rushed. I wanted to be able to ask as many questions as I wanted about my treatment. I wanted to feel as though there were no stupid questions.

7. *I kept a binder to help me keep track of all my paperwork.* Actually, I didn't do this right away, but I wish I had. It sounds so obvious to keep a binder, but I was in denial that I would have so much material pertaining to my cancer treatment. I bought a black three-ring binder to hold every blood test, insurance form, various letters, hospital information, and of course blank loose-leaf paper for notes. I put it in a carryall bag and would take it like a briefcase to every appointment.

8. *If I was unhappy at any office, I could leave.* Okay, I'll elaborate. If I was waiting in a doctor's office and it was overcrowded, the staff was unfriendly, or the wait was more than three hours, no matter how good the doctor

was, I knew that place was not for me. I always knew in the back of my mind that if a doctor was not a match for me, I had the ability to get up and leave.

9. *I could stop treatment.* I made a decision early on to take each day as it came. If I decided to go with traditional chemotherapy and the doctor prescribed eight chemotherapy sessions, but I decided it was pure hell after the fourth treatment, I would stop. I was the one in charge of my health, and only I could determine if I wanted to continue. If my body was telling me "enough," then I would listen. I kept in mind that as the CEO, I could fire anyone at any time!

Chapter 4

My Version of Cut, Poison, and Burn

Part 1: Cut—Surgery

I made my second decision as CEO of my body to go ahead with a lumpectomy to remove the lump in my breast. I didn't really think twice about setting up the surgery, since removing the mass that had the potential to spread made sense to me. Frank and I read the statistics behind the procedure, and it seemed like a no-brainer. The surgery was scheduled for three weeks later. I used that time to rearrange any commitments that I had and spend time with my family. I also prepared my body for what was ahead. I continued to stay physically fit, eat healthy meals, and drink plenty of water.

I had to do presurgical testing before the surgery could be performed. Frank came with me and helped me fill out the stack of paperwork. My presurgical testing included an interview with an RN at the hospital, an EKG, and, of course, my favorite: a blood draw. I met with an RN named Kathy in the presurgical testing department. She gave me details about the surgery, plus parking instructions, and advised me to wear a zip-up shirt the day of surgery. She also told me to wear cotton underpants so I could keep them on during surgery; otherwise I would be completely naked.

When I set out on my cancer journey, I put out to the universe that I wanted to encounter as many nice, helpful, friendly people as I could and I did! I tried to attract them especially when I felt nervous or upset about a medical procedure. In those moments, I made an extra effort to be super nice and friendly to the person who was helping me.

I would bring silly stickers with me to doctors' offices or the hospital and give them out as special prizes. I know it sounds really goofy, but people really appreciated it when I would go out of my way to say thank you.

The lumpectomy was to be performed at a local hospital in their ambulatory center, which meant I would have surgery and be home the same day. The surgery was pretty straightforward and routine. Dr. McCloy would cut out the small cancer mass in my left breast and the surrounding tissue in an attempt to get any stray cancer cells that could be in the area. In reviewing the procedure, Dr. McCloy explained that I might wake up with a drain near my breast area. If the sentinel node, which is the main lymph node in the breast, tested positive for cancer cells, then the surrounding lymph nodes would need to be removed in case the cancer had spread to them and throughout the rest of my body. If lymph nodes needed to be removed, a drain would be placed to help my body adapt to the missing lymph nodes. None of the doctors I interviewed thought my sentinel node would be affected. My fear was that I would wake up without a left breast, but Dr. McCloy assured me that was not going to happen.

THE RED STRING STORY

I was confident in my decision with my surgeon, and I was drinking more water and practicing breathing techniques all in preparation for my surgery, but I wanted to add more. I called my friend Maureen Calamia, who is a Feng Shui consultant, to see if there were any extra rituals I could do to ensure good health.

Maureen recommended a Chinese ritual called the Red String. I purchased an eighteen-inch red string, and nine days prior to my surgery I cut it in half. One half stayed with me, and the other half went to Frank. We each kept the ribbon on us for all nine days prior to surgery. Frank kept his in his pants pocket, and I kept mine in my bra. On the day of my surgery, Frank had his piece in his pocket and mine was tied to my hospital bracelet.

The premise behind this ritual was that it encouraged good fortune in health or for someone with an illness. The cutting of the string represented our ability to be connected even when we were apart. We did this ritual three separate times throughout my cancer journey. Having the ribbon on my hospital bracelet created a conversation with others and helped calm me the day of my surgery.

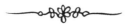

THE MORNING OF MY SURGERY I got up, showered with antibacterial soap, and put on my cotton underwear that the hospital suggested I wear. We left the house by five thirty and drove traffic-free for the next thirty minutes. I drove to the hospital because driving calms me down. We sat in silence and listened to music that I picked, which meant me flipping through all the radio stations ranging from spa to rock.

We pulled up to the hospital ambulatory center and checked in. We waited about ten minutes before I was called to change into hospital garb. My clothes went into a locker to which Frank kept the key. I wore a gown that opened in the front (as if there was any other way anymore) and was put into a nice private room to wait. It was a comfy room with privacy blinds, a TV, a reclining chair for me, and a chair for Frank. I was more anxious about the IV than the surgery, because I knew I would be awake for the IV placement. I met with a really nice nurse whom I told straight off the bat that my blood pressure was high and I was nervous about the needle. The IV went in without a hitch. I waited for the various "players" to parade in: the anesthesiologist, the surgical and presurgical nurses, and the surgeon.

Frank brought the iPad, and we occupied our time by watching comedies. Our favorite show to watch was reruns of *Arrested Development*, which made us laugh and distracted us from what was about to happen. Plus, the hospital staff got a kick walking into my room and finding us laughing hysterically.

The surgery had several steps, starting with Dr. McCloy drawing on my left breast with a black marker to indicate where the mass was located. Then, there was the placement of a guide wire, surgery to remove the mass, and testing the sentinel node to see if the cancer had spread. Depending on the results of the sentinel node biopsy, more lymph nodes might be removed immediately.

I was extremely anxious as I was wheeled upstairs to the mammogram area. I probably should have requested some meds to relax me, but I didn't want the extra drugs in my system. I was already going to have enough between the anesthesia and pain meds.

Now, imagine me sitting in a wheelchair wrapped in blankets to stay warm, parked in the hallway in front of the mammogram room. I was visibly upset because I was about to undergo surgery for freaking breast cancer. Suddenly, a woman approached me from out of nowhere and handed me a large canvas bag. It was imprinted with pink ribbons and full of breast cancer pamphlets and booklets. I looked at this woman like she was crazy. I can't even recall what she said to me, because I was stunned that I was being approached as I was waiting to go in for surgery. I remember looking at her like she had three heads. The incident pushed me over the edge, and I lost it. I felt like I had been dealing well with the impending surgery so far, but to then have this cancer bag put right in my face was just unthinkable. I fell apart, sobbing. Frank stepped in and took the bag from the woman, because I would not look up and make eye contact with her. The last thing I needed that day was breast cancer support stuff. I needed to stay focused and get through surgery. Literally, I took it one step at a time. If I needed any of that paraphernalia after surgery, I knew where to look. But I'm so grateful that Frank had the wherewithal to make sure I never saw that bag again.

When it was time to leave for the surgery, I don't remember anything other than walking from the wheelchair to the surgical table. I talked with the surgical nurses about what music I preferred during surgery. The next thing I remember is waking up in the recovery room.

I heard things going on within the recovery room, but I wasn't fully present. I overheard nurses saying Dr. McCloy needed to talk with Christine before she could see her husband. I waited for what seemed like an hour. Dr. McCloy had to finish another surgery before she could talk to me. I was prepared for the worst. I just kept remembering Dr. McCloy telling me she would not remove my breast. I was slowly coming around mentally and physically, and I saw that I had a clear plastic tube next to me on the hospital bed. I figured it was the dreaded drain. Somehow at that moment I was not too scared. I was alive, wasn't in pain, and figured I could handle whatever came next.

The nurses wheeled me back into the "private waiting room" at the ambulatory center, and I waited for Dr. McCloy to talk to me. I started to feel anxious at this point. My mind wandered to thoughts that the cancer had spread to my bones and brain. I was waiting alone, without Frank by my side. I wondered why she needed to talk to me without Frank. When Dr. McCloy arrived about ten minutes later, she told me she had removed the mass. The tissue in the surrounding area looked good, but the sentinel node tested positive for cancer cells, and she had removed eight lymph nodes in my left arm. We would have to wait a few days for the test results to see if the cancer had spread to any of the other lymph nodes, which meant the cancer could have spread to other parts of my body.

I remained calm and thought, *Okay, I can do this.*

I wasn't panicked, but I was sad that my story couldn't end here. I knew that more cancer treatment was in my future now. I wasn't thinking about death per se. I knew deep down I was going to be fine. I was unnerved that Frank was still not with me. Where the hell was Frank?

Dr. McCloy explained to me when she gave Frank the news that the cancer might have spread, he took it very badly. She told him to go outside and breathe some fresh air. I think the idea that the cancer was worse than we thought was just more than Frank could handle. He had been so strong and optimistic until then. In short, it rocked his world. But I really wanted to see him. When Dr. McCloy finally brought him to my room, we cried together, thinking that the cancer might have spread beyond the original little mass. We were unsure what the future held for us.

We waited in our private room mourning the situation. I wasn't ready to leave the hospital just yet, even though I was ready to be discharged. We stayed in our room wrapping our heads around what had happened. Was the cancer throughout my body? I hadn't thought about what this diagnosis really meant (even in retrospect). I started preparing myself to go from thinking I would get away with just radiation treatment to the unthinkable addition of chemotherapy. I was sad that this freaking cancer journey might be extended.

After about an hour of sitting in that little room with the blinds drawn, we got ourselves emotionally together. Physically, I was fine. I wasn't in any post-surgery pain. I was a little thrown by the plastic tube coming out of the side of my body, but somehow after receiving my new potential diagnosis, the drain seemed manageable. I pinned the drain to the inside of my zip-up sweat jacket, so it was completely hidden. (Yet another great tip: wear a zip-up sweatshirt with pockets.) I was able to get myself dressed, clean my face, and appear fine for my kids. Frank drove home that afternoon. I said hi to the kids so they could see me, and then I climbed into bed and zoned out for a few hours. We did not share the news from the surgery with the kids.

When I woke up, it was dinnertime and the kids really wanted to spend time with me. The last thing I wanted was to climb out of bed and socialize, but I also knew it was exactly what I needed. I joined the family downstairs at the dining room table and ate food from our favorite organic restaurant. I enjoyed half of an organic burger with salad and felt so much better after eating and talking with my family. I was emotionally exhausted, and I'm sure having all those drugs in my system wasn't helping.

POST SURGERY SELF-CARE

Dr. McCloy called the next day to see how I was feeling. I felt fine, except that my left breast was swollen. I told her it was a little odd having one breast bigger than the other, but I was really trying to go with it. I had some bruising, but nothing too bad. I put ice on my left breast, and kept my bra on for support and to help prevent scarring.

Over the next few days we weren't thinking about the impending test results to see if cancer was present in the other lymph nodes. We were dealing with the task at hand—recovering from surgery and dealing with the drain. The whole thought that a fist-size, plastic bubble attached to a twelve-inch-long plastic tube was coming out of my body totally freaked me out. I was not capable of emptying the fluid from the drain right after surgery, so I asked for help. Frank emptied the fluid from the drain into a container and recorded the liquid measurements several times a day. When Frank was not around, I asked my nurse friends (Mary or Margaret) to help me. For the next three days I received help emptying the drain. I was thankful that I could put the drain out of my mind and rely on others to take care of me when I needed it. Eventually, I came around and wasn't so grossed out by the idea of emptying it.

I remembered my midwife telling me after my children were born that your body has only one chance to physically heal. I wanted my body to heal from the surgery and recover from the trauma and the drugs used during the surgery.

So I stayed on task with my one big job: letting my body heal from the surgery. This task helped ease my mind as I waited for the test results. Although I did not take any additional pain medication, lots of drugs were left in my system from the surgery, so I wanted to be sure I detoxified. I drank tons of water and enlisted friends to make body-cleansing teas for me. My friend and fellow health coach Tina Annibell would make a large thermos for me with dandelion, nettle, licorice, milk thistle, burdock root, ginger, and cinnamon. This tea was made with loose tea leaves, but many premade detox teas are also available. I probably drank close to thirty-two ounces of water plus another thirty-two ounces of tea for at least two days. It seemed like I did nothing more than sleep, drink, and eat for the next week.

I also tried different healing modalities, including energy work like Reiki and reflexology. I was new to Reiki, but I knew other friends of mine had tried it and raved about how their body and mind felt afterward. I also read about it in various healing-arts books and heard it was perfect for people recovering from surgery because it's not a true hands-on treatment like massage. Reiki is a Japanese technique for stress reduction and relaxation that also promotes healing. It's based on the idea that an unseen "life force energy" flows through us and that "laying hands" on a person can promote healing.

Reflexology is the practice of applying pressure to the feet, hands, or ears with specific techniques without the use of lotions. These pressure points can effect physical changes in the body. For example, the area around your ankles has an energy link to your liver. Liver is the organ used to detoxify things from your body. I wanted my liver to help me detoxify all the drugs that were given to me during the surgery. I knew after surgery my body was sore, and I really wanted a form of relaxation that would make me feel better.

My friend Nancy is a Reiki and reflexology therapist, so she seemed like the perfect person to try it out with. After the hour with her, I felt much better. It was an opportunity for my body to heal on another level. Reflexology and Reiki both helped my mind and body relax after the surgery.

I watched comedies to help me laugh each day. I rested and stayed in bed for hours. I went for short walks in the woods. I ate green salads and warming homemade soups, and included small amounts of organic red meat to help my body recover faster. I practiced what I like to call ultimate self-care. I wanted to show respect to my body and prepare it for what might lie ahead.

The phone rang four days later with results of the lymph node test. Dr. McCloy told me all the lymph nodes tested negative; the cancer had not spread throughout my body. *Wow*—some really good news! I felt relieved on one hand, but still scared because cancer had still spread to at least one lymph node. (Remember, the main lymph node, the sentinel node, did test positive for cancer cells.) I would have to wait a few more weeks to get the full pathology report from the oncologist. I continued waiting and recovering.

I remember telling Frank the great news that the cancer had not spread, and we were both relieved and, of course, happy. But we also thought, *Okay, we got past one hurdle.* Many more hurdles were still ahead. You'd think we would have had a party to celebrate the great news we had received so far, but we didn't. I couldn't look at a calendar, never mind make any plans, because I just didn't know what was going to happen to me. We were still waiting for the dreaded visit with the oncologist. We knew that the sentinel node testing positive was a real game changer in my cancer treatment, and neither of us was ready to hear what Dr. V had to say.

Within a week the swelling in my left breast had lessened. But even today the left breast is slightly larger than the right one! How funny is that? My surgeon explained that this is normal because of adhesions near the surgery site. The size difference is not really visible unless you look closely. My image of myself had changed at this point; I was so happy with what I saw. I felt truly grateful for my body and all that it had done for me. I was a little angry with myself for not truly appreciating it until this moment. I was just so happy to be alive and to have the cancer out of my body.

I was so concerned (and rightfully so) about getting the cancer out that I really hadn't thought about the recovery process. I missed my exercise. Exercise had always helped me clear my mind, and although I was walking in the woods with the dog, it wasn't helping my arm.

But about four weeks after my surgery, my breast was still swollen and bruised, and I had limited arm movement. I felt a strange pulling sensation from deep within my arm. I felt this deep pulling sensation as a result of the tendons that were cut during surgery. It felt like extremely tight strings in my armpit area kept me from moving my left arm above my head. I did the exercises that Dr. McCloy instructed me to do, which included stretching, but I kept thinking, *Will I ever be the same again?*

Since running and kickboxing were out of the question, I turned back to yoga. In the past, going to hot yoga had been something on my to-do list, but I had never made the time to go. Now I knew the added heat of the yoga room would help me stretch my arm. I went to the warm (90-degree) yoga classes first to get my body adjusted to the heat. After seeing the benefits of the warm yoga, I decided to try the hot yoga, where the temperature in the room gets to 120 degrees.

After just four classes, my arm was able to move like normal again. I had full range of motion and the tugging feeling was gone. I worked on poses that opened my chest area. I attended classes that closed with a meditation. I was working not only on my body, but on my mind too. In each class, I tried to keep my focus on the task at hand and not think about the past or the future. I would think only about the pose I was doing right then and there. I tried to take that thought process back into the rest of my life too. It was a struggle to maintain that mind-set of just "being." But I came across a quote from Deepak Chopra that helped. He says, "We are human beings, not human doers." I liked the mental and physical results that yoga gave me, and I truly believe that the yoga helped me recover fully.

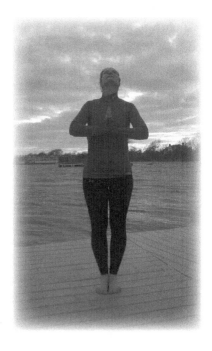

Yoga helps me stretch my arm and relax me.

My surgeon, Dr. McCloy, recommended I wear a comfortable bra 24/7. As uncomfortable as that sounds, it was not so bad. My breasts were all contained in one area and lifted. Dr. McCloy explained that the bra helped keep the breast tissue from scarring. The bra kept the breasts up, preventing gravity from pulling them down and creating more problems.

My breasts also felt very full and voluptuous. I didn't feel like something had been taken out of my breast; I felt like something was added. It was a nice feeling, which was such a surprise to me. I felt sexy after my surgery. There, I said it. The fullness of my breast was reminiscent of when my milk came in after the babies were born, although back then, both breasts were enlarged, and this time only my left breast was enlarged! The drain inserted in my armpit area did not make me feel sexy, but as I said, I enlisted help with it until I was able to manage it on my own.

I continued with my job of healing my body. During my healing process I cooked most of my own foods at home. Homemade soups with various beans, greens, and root vegetables became a staple. I experimented with green smoothies with the intention of adding as many healthy greens into my body as possible. I learned during my nutrition studies that green leafy vegetables are powerful antioxidants and could help my body fight cancer cells. I added green veggies along with fruits into smoothies to boost my immunity. I continued to experiment with which smoothies tasted good and continued researching healing foods for myself.

Whatever I was doing was working, because I felt great, my skin was glowing, and my energy level was good—so good that most of my friends didn't even know I had cancer.

What I Did to Help My Body Recover from Surgery:

1. **I rested, rested, and then rested some more.** I made it my job to stay in bed and rest. I knew that my body had been through an emotional and physical upheaval and that I had only one opportunity to heal from this surgery.

2. **I drank, drank, and then drank some more.** My body was not used to all the drugs I was given at the hospital, and I wanted them flushed out of my system. Plus, water helps your tissues heal.

3. **I watched comedies to keep my spirits up.** If I wasn't sleeping, I was resting in bed while watching funny shows. Fun, lighthearted, thirty-minute episodes helped me stay positive and helped me stay in bed to rest.

4. **I added green leafy veggies to every meal.** I slowly started crowding out packaged foods and including more greens with my meals. If I was making soup, I added chopped greens. If I was making a shake, I added a handful of spinach.

5. **I added yoga to help my arm recover.** Once I was given the okay from my surgeon to stretch my arm, I started slowly at home and then added yoga to my weekly routine.

6. **I walked in nature.** Every morning I took my dog Zoe to my local nature trail for a thirty-minute walk. My walk helped me stay focused on what was around me. I would search for turtles, listen for birds, and just enjoy the tall green trees around me.

TEST RESULTS: PATHOLOGY REPORT

After waiting six weeks, my results came in. Frank and I went to the oncologist's office to find out my next course of treatment. Frank and I didn't discuss out loud what the next steps would be. We started our own research. We each read as many cancer books as we could emotionally handle. I left Frank in charge of really researching the details of chemotherapy. Now, mind you, the idea of chemotherapy had been in the back of my mind since finding out about the diagnosis, but I truly tried to take it one step at a time and put it out of my mind.

I was sick to my stomach driving to the office, wondering if the doctor was going to recommend the dreaded chemotherapy. I was very quiet and kept to myself, holding back the urge to burst out in tears any second. My visit to this office was similar to the previous time I had been there: lab stop (with finger prick), then vitals taken. Fortunately, no blood draw was needed.

Before the surgery when I interviewed various surgeons, all of them thought I would just need a lumpectomy and radiation. In my mind these two courses of action seemed very doable. They made sense to me—cut out the cancer and then radiate the breast to kill any leftover cells. So much evidence backed up the effectiveness of radiation that although I didn't like it, I understood the necessity of it. But having the sentinel lymph node test positive for cancer cells was a game changer. I was about to find out how much so.

My oncologist used two major tests to determine the next course of treatment. The first one was the BRACCA test. This is a genetic test to see if I carried the so-called breast cancer gene. I decided to do this because I felt a responsibility to my daughter, Emily. That test came back negative; I did not carry the gene, although carrying it would not have meant that Emily would automatically get breast cancer.

The other test is called the Oncotype DX test. This is a relatively new test from a California company that looks at your actual pathology and determines the probability of cancer coming back. This test revealed that I had a relatively low chance of the cancer returning. But, based on my young age of forty-two and the fact that there were cancer cells (although low grade) present in the sentinel node, the oncologist still recommended that I do the chemotherapy. After my oncologist reviewed the results with us, he just assumed that I would sign up right then and there for the chemotherapy, but instead I left the office to think about my next steps.

I knew going into this cancer adventure that the oncologist I had chosen was very conservative and did not believe in any other type of cancer treatments than chemotherapy and radiation. I did not attempt to change his thoughts; after all, that's what he had studied and practiced for twenty years. My point of view was not about to change any of that. I respected all my doctors' opinions. I always listened to what they said, and then researched on my own and came up with the treatment that was right for me.

I reminded myself that the oncologist I was with treated thousands of patients. He used statistics and "playing the numbers," which allowed him to save more lives. For an individual like myself, patient statistics were meaningless. I wanted to find a doctor who would not lump me into a large statistical group. I wanted someone to treat me for me.

The idea of chemotherapy for my cancer just didn't sit with me. I was feeling healthy, exercising, eating well, and looking great. I couldn't wrap my head around the idea of putting the chemotherapy poison into my system to make me well. I knew deep down I would not follow that course of treatment.

On the drive home, Frank and I tried to celebrate the fact that my Oncotype DX test came back with a low recurrence rate and that I didn't carry the breast cancer gene. We were happy and relieved that my cancer was at a low stage 2. I so wanted to enjoy the good news and stop there. We should have been jumping for joy at another great test result! But when the doctor told me he felt I could benefit greatly from chemo, it took the air out of my balloon. I was just not ready to face the fact that the chemotherapy drugs could help me stay cancer-free.

PART 2: POISON—INSULIN POTENTIATION THERAPY

I knew other options for cancer therapy were out there. I watched documentaries, researched online, and talked with other cancer patients. One type of alternative cancer treatment that Frank and I investigated was called Insulin Potentiation Therapy (IPT). The therapy uses insulin, and takes advantage of the powerful, cell-killing effects of ordinary chemotherapy drugs used in very low doses.

Here's a little more background on IPT from www.Linchitzwellness. com:

> Cancer cells get their energy by secreting their own insulin, and they stimulate themselves to grow by secreting their own insulin-like growth factor (IGF). These are their mechanisms of malignancy. Insulin and IGF work by attaching to special cell membrane receptors, and these receptors are sixteen times more concentrated on cancer cell membranes than on normal cells. These receptors are the key to IPT. Using insulin in IPT, the low dose chemotherapy gets channeled specifically inside the cancer cells, killing them more effectively, and with minimal chemotherapy side effects.
>
> Insulin Potentiation Therapy was developed in Mexico by a family of physicians—Drs. Donato, Perez, Garcia. During the last twenty-five years they and other doctors have collaborated with their Mexican colleagues to provide a sound scientific basis for

the therapy, and getting documentation of this published in the scientific medical literature. Their common goal has always been, and yet remains, to get IPT properly studied in this country so greater numbers of physicians and patients in the United States could use it. An in vitro study at Georgetown University showed insulin increases the penetration of chemotherapy into cancer cells ten-thousand-fold. Another study from Uruguay on chemotherapy-resistant patients (treatment failures) showed shrinkage of tumors when the patients were then treated with IPT.

I heard about an IPT doctor from a local news documentary and kept his name in the back of my head with the intention of giving it out to anyone looking for alternative cancer treatments. I never thought I might need his name myself. Coincidentally, a RN friend of mine (Peggy) attended a lecture given by the same doctor in the documentary and raved about what he had to say. This IPT doctor was only one hour away from my home, so I called to make an appointment. I researched Dr. Linchitz and learned that he had graduated from Cornell University Medical College and completed his residency at the University of California, San Francisco. He is board certified by the American Board of Psychiatry and Neurology and has a variety of other board certifications as well. But what I didn't learn until I met him was that he too had had cancer—and like me, for no apparent reason. He had been given a diagnosis of lung cancer, having never smoked a day in his life. He was also in excellent health as a competitive triathlete and led a healthy lifestyle, yet he was given a 50 percent chance to live.

Although IPT is not a "medically accepted" form of cancer treatment, it made sense to us. I would be getting the chemo drugs, but the drugs would target the cancer cells in a way that was different from traditional chemotherapy. We fully understood that there was limited scientific evidence behind IPT. But Frank and I also understood what it took to get a scientific study published. Most scientific studies are funded by drug companies, and unfortunately no drug company was going to fund a study that suggested using 10 percent of their drug.

I knew this office operated differently when the doctor himself called me to talk about my specific cancer before I even came into the office.

Dr. Linchitz explained what reports to bring and said he had successfully treated women with breast cancer.

Frank and I went to see him in late March. It was raining, and the drive to his office felt long. The office was in an area we were not that familiar with, so the GPS came in handy. Neither one of us spoke much on the way. We were each in our own mind. I had control of the radio, because it always helped calm me down. In my mind we were just going there to gather information. We were just gathering facts about another form of treatment.

The office looked similar to a regular doctor's office. It was a multi-doctor practice in a regular office building, but the energy felt very different. It was a little calmer, and the people who worked there were extremely friendly. Lavender essential oils were diffused in the waiting room. Although lavender is a very calming oil, I still felt super nervous. I had to fill out the same type of medical health history forms. I asked Frank to fill them out so I could practice my deep abdominal relaxation breathing. I tried to occupy myself with the health magazines while we waited twenty minutes. We were the first appointment of the day, so the waiting room was empty; we were not surrounded by other patients.

Dr. Linchitz greeted us. He was dressed very conservatively and wore a long white lab coat. He was very much like every other doctor I visited except we talked for about an hour before he even did a physical exam. He wanted to know everything about me before cancer and what had I done so far to treat it. He reviewed the test results and other information we had brought with us: my blood tests, my pathology results, and information about my overall health. We sat on the other side of the desk as I told my cancer story thus far. He asked us, "Why are you here?"

Why were we there? It was a really good question. I was there to have this doctor tell me I was a healthy individual who would be fine without any treatment. I wanted him to tell me I could go along my merry way. I am not joking here. I really hoped this doctor was going to give me a "cancer pass." I truly thought my healthy lifestyle would give me an exemption.

I was devastated when he explained how I could benefit from Insulin Potentiation Therapy. I just started bawling my eyes out right then and there. I had been numb about cancer treatment up until this point. I thought somehow in the back of my mind I was going to get out of it. Of course, I could choose to do nothing, but talking with him made me realize I needed to do some form of chemotherapy.

Not only was Dr. Linchitz talking about the low-dose chemo (IPT), but he also explained the benefits of having a "portacath" surgically inserted into my body so the chemotherapy could be administered easily. I told him about my fear of IV needles. This discussion was way more than I could handle. The tears started rolling down my face. My shirt was soaked with sweat, and my head was pounding. I wanted to run away.

The next thing I knew, Frank was helping me get up from Dr. Linchitz's private office to get some blood work done. If I was going to receive IPT at this office, some more testing had to take place. Although I was still unsure about my next steps, I went ahead with the blood work.

As we walked down the hall to the treatment room, I couldn't stop crying. Reality had set in that I needed some form of chemotherapy treatment. I was still unsure which kind of treatment, but with stage 2 cancer, I felt I had to do something.

The nurse quickly and adeptly took blood from my arm (ten vials' worth) and showed me a brochure of what the portacath looked like. I was not capable of taking in the information. I remember literally turning my head away from the booklet. Not only was Dr. Linchitz not giving me the cancer pass I'd thought I was going to get, but he also thought I would benefit from treatment and needed a "piece" surgically inserted.

Frank drove on the way home because I could not stop crying. I confessed to him that I had thought Dr. Linchitz would tell me I didn't need treatment. The look on Frank's face showed such compassion for me. He said he wished he had known what was going on in my head, because he would have prepared me better for the office visit.

As for next steps, no decisions had to be made just yet. I sat quietly with my options: "proven" traditional chemotherapy treatment with many potential side effects, low-dose chemotherapy (IPT) "unproven within the medical community" with little to no side effects, or nothing at all.

After much thought and discussion with Frank and close friends, I committed to the IPT treatment and the port placement. I felt that I needed to do some kind of treatment that would kill off any cancer cells that were floating around in my body. The decision to go ahead with the

IPT by this point seemed like the lesser of two evils. I would receive the benefits of chemotherapy, but at a dosage that was not going to make me sick or leave me with long-term health issues. I felt like it was a decision I could live with.

Dr. Linchitz ordered different tests than a conventional oncologist. The big test I agreed to was to have my actual pathology from the lumpectomy sent to Germany. My sample would be tested against various chemotherapy drugs to see which one would work best at killing my specific cancer. This "alternative" test is not offered here in the States and we paid $4,000 out of pocket for it, but it made sense to us. If I was going to do chemotherapy, I wanted to be sure I got the right drug for me, not just the standard drug for all breast cancer patients. I felt like I had found the doctor who would treat me and my cancer.

14 vs. 20: How Much Chemo Did I Agree To?

When I went back to review my test results from Dr. Linchitz, I went alone. Frank had a prior commitment, and I was feeling stronger about my decision to go ahead with IPT. Dr. Linchitz reviewed the test results from Germany with me and got me set up for my IPT appointments. He said in passing something about twenty treatments. I said, "What? Twenty treatments!" I explained that when Frank and I had come in for the consultation, we had each written down that I would receive fourteen IPT treatments. "Where did we get the fourteen treatments?" Dr. Linchitz very calmly said that twenty treatments was the standard. He was unsure where Frank and I had gotten fourteen, but we must have heard fourteen for a reason. He then suggested that I complete fourteen treatments, if that was what my intuition was telling me. How empowered I felt! I committed 100 percent right there and then to finishing fourteen IPT treatments. My IPT schedule started with treatment twice a week for four weeks, then once a week for four weeks, finishing with treatment once every other week for two weeks, giving me a total of fourteen IPT treatments.

PREPPING FOR TREATMENT

Although I wasn't happy about having more surgery, my nurse friends explained the benefits of the portacath. One of the big benefits was avoiding constantly accessing my blood via IV needle in my arm or hand. Yes, even after all these months, I was still afraid of needles in my arm. My friends understood my fear and told me I could avoid all that by having the port put into my chest, and that doing so would keep my veins healthy. The chemotherapy drugs tend to "harden" the veins even in low doses, which in turn can make them more difficult to access later in treatment. One of the worst-case scenarios, my nurse friends explained, was going in for my treatment and the nurse being unable to access a vein. The prospect of having to endure pain scared me, and so did the thought of extending treatment.

I finally read the brochure for the portacath, and it was described as a small medical appliance installed beneath the skin. The catheter connects the port to a vein and is used to administer medication. Picture having a small, metal disk about the size of a quarter placed inside your body. This idea was beyond my wildest nightmares. Not only had I agreed to get the IPT, but I also agreed to go under the knife again to have this foreign object put into my body. Who had I become?

The port was placed halfway between my collarbone and the top of my right breast. It was put on the right side because I couldn't have anything "done" to the left side because of the removal of my lymph nodes.

My surgeon, Dr. McCloy, put my portacath in for me at the same ambulatory center where my lumpectomy took place. The procedure was supposed to take a quick thirty minutes and then I would go home. I scheduled to be the first surgery of the morning, knowing Frank would take me to the hospital and then home so he could still make it to work by twelve thirty.

The quick thirty minutes turned into three hours. Dr. McCloy did not like the angle of my vein near the port, so a vascular surgeon needed to be brought in to assist. All I can say in retrospect is poor Frank. Can you imagine him sitting there waiting for me to come out of this "simple" surgery within thirty minutes and then not hearing word from the surgeon until three hours later?

I didn't know any of this until later in the day when Frank and Dr. McCloy explained it all afterward. The port did get placed and I was not in any medical danger. I didn't have much post-surgery pain, but I was tired from all the medication I had been given. We made it home just in time for Frank to go to work. I climbed into bed and slept the rest of the day. The kids were being entertained by a "kid-sitter."

I left the bandage in place, because the thought of this device being inside me freaked me out. I was not ready to look at the "bump" underneath my skin. The port was placed on Thursday, and I went for my first IPT treatment on Monday.

The idea that I could physically feel this port in this sensitive, unfleshy part of my body reminded me that I was a cancer patient after all. Any other cancer person who sees this scar on my body will know it's a port scar. Port scar = cancer.

IPT Treatment 1

My first IPT treatment started with the one-hour drive to Dr. Linchitz's office. Frank was by my side. I took the first appointment of the morning. I liked doing it first thing for several reasons. One, traffic is a little lighter at six in the morning. Two, I needed to fast for the treatment, and I knew I would be hungry. Plus, I liked having the afternoon to rest.

Dr. Linchitz had assigned his head nurse, Marybeth, to me, because of my obvious anxiety about starting my IPT journey. Marybeth had called me a few days earlier to review the treatment and explained that I needed to bring fruit and protein with me. My big question was how was I going to feel after treatment? Was I going to be sick, tired, or overall miserable? Marybeth assured me that I would be able to handle the treatment just fine and that if I didn't, they could prescribe medicine and/or herbal remedies to help me through my treatments. I was also really scared about the needle used to access my port. Marybeth didn't discount my fears. Instead she prescribed a topical numbing cream for me to use on the skin over my port.

When Frank and I got to the office, I really had no idea what to expect. I was shown on paper what was going to happen (because you sign your life away) and reviewed the treatment with Marybeth, but fully understanding what was going to happen to me physically was something else.

We went into the treatment area, and my regular vitals—weight, blood pressure, and heart rate—were taken. I started tearing up and couldn't talk, because I was on the verge of a major meltdown. I was thinking about the toxic chemicals that were about to enter my body. I was also fearful that the treatment might hurt. This was the journey I did not want to take, a journey I thought I would never have to take. I still couldn't believe I had cancer. I could not face that fact, even as I was sitting getting ready to have chemotherapy drugs put into my body.

I was reclined in a dark brown leather chair surrounded by three young female nurses in hospital scrubs. My body was in a strangely semi-relaxed state, and I had a clear tube, twenty-four inches long, coming out of the upper right side of my chest. I could hear people talking to me, but it sounded more like mumbled background noise. The only words I could hear were the ones playing in my head. The sounds were from the eighties band the Talking Heads. I imagined hearing the following words repeated with a funky beat:

> "You may ask yourself, well, how did I get here?
> You may ask yourself, am I right, am I wrong?
> You may say to yourself, my God, what have I done?"

That song played in my head over and over as my brand new port was used to inject medicine into my body. The port access gave Marybeth a bit of a problem, as she had a little difficulty feeling for the flat part of my port. Although I had my numbing cream on, I could still feel the pressure, and my anxiety level went through the roof.

Tears were streaming down my face, my shirt was drenched in sweat, and my palms were wet. (I am sweating right now just thinking back to that day.) Once she found the port, the rest seemed easier. Blood was drawn from the port, which was a highlight for me. No more getting poked in the arm for a blood draw!

The following premeds were administered through the port, and my body did not have any adverse reactions:

- Decadron for reducing the severity of any allergic reaction that might occur
- Toradol for pain prevention

- Heparin for reducing clot formation
- Zofran for nausea

The next step was the insulin. My fasting blood sugar level was taken and recorded. Then came a dose of insulin through my port line. We (Marybeth, Frank, and myself) waited for my blood glucose level to drop to a "therapeutic level" so the chemotherapy drugs could be administered.

Marybeth explained to me that different people have different reactions when their blood sugar levels drop. She stayed by my side and checked my blood every thirty seconds via a finger prick to monitor my blood sugar levels. My reaction when my blood sugar level dropped was one of pure relaxation. Finally, a good side effect! Marybeth knew my levels were within "therapeutic range" because I seemed very relaxed and paused my nonstop babbling.

The three different fluorescent yellow chemotherapy IV bags were inserted into my port line. The colors of these IV bags looked as though they would sting when they entered my body, but they didn't. I felt fine after the chemotherapy drugs went into my system. Another happy surprise!

When it was time for me to raise my blood glucose levels, I drank some fruit juice, ate a banana, and then ate an apple with almond butter. After a few minutes of eating and drinking, my finger was pricked again to be sure my blood glucose levels had risen to within normal range. My levels were good, so I was allowed to eat my bean salad for protein, which would help stabilize my blood sugar levels without additional medications. The treatment was almost finished with another IV bag of medicine to help flush my body of toxins. I called this the pee medicine, because it made me get up and urinate every fifteen minutes or so. It was fine by me. I liked the idea of my body ridding itself of the unused medicine.

Last, I got hooked up to a high dose of IV vitamin C. Vitamin C therapy is yet another "alternative" cancer treatment. Studies have shown that high doses of vitamin C (25–100 grams), when given intravenously, have the potential to destroy cancer cells while leaving healthy cells alone.

After my first treatment, Frank and I walked back to the car together. I felt deeply relaxed. Frank drove home, and I asked him if Marybeth had slipped me something to relax me. He assured me she hadn't. My feeling of relaxation was just my body's response to finishing the first treatment. I understood now how much worry and fear I had been holding on to. Now that the first treatment was complete, I knew I was doing the right type of treatment for me.

Tears of relief streamed down my face. (I'm an equal opportunity crier.) I was glad to be doing something active about my cancer treatment. The time and energy that I had put into researching which treatment was best for me had finally been put into play. I was doing something about the cancer and about future prevention. The surgery seemed necessary to me—remove something that was cancerous and had the potential to grow. But it seemed easy to me, and I could wrap my mind around it. The IPT was something else. I clung onto that good feeling on a physical level as well as an emotional level. The relief I felt knowing that I could go ahead with this treatment without losing my hair or being sick was just overwhelming. I had long hair already, but since I was going to be able to keep it, I decided to keep growing it out.

When I returned home, I just climbed into bed and rested. Even though I felt fine physically, my emotional state had worn me out. I wanted to rest and let the medicine do its stuff. I rested for a while, and then went downstairs to make myself a shake. Dr. Linchitz gave me a packaged, powdered mix that consisted of dried mushrooms, herbs, amino acids, and B vitamins to help my body heal from treatment. The shakes were easy to mix, and once I added frozen berries, they tasted just fine.

One Major Setback

I awoke on Friday after my IPT to a swollen right forearm. Now, remember, I had had the lymph nodes removed on my left side and was told to look out for lymphedema. Lymphedema is when the lymphatic fluid in your body does not flow properly and causes swelling. But because it was on my right side, I was really confused.

My arm felt stiff. The skin felt warm and tight. I knew something was wrong. I showed Frank, and he was very concerned too. *Oh no!* I thought. This fear wasn't just in my mind. Frank could see that something was not right with my arm and was taking it seriously. He called the surgeon for me, because I became a real basket case. I tried to relax, but was unable to quiet my mind. When he got ahold of Dr. McCloy, she said it sounded like a blood clot caused by the port.

Oh my God! I had freaking cancer, and now I am going to die of a blood clot was all I could think.

Dr. McCloy sent me to the radiologist's office for a sonogram of my chest and arm to try to figure out if I did indeed have a blood clot. Frank had work, and I couldn't ask him to cancel his day filled with patients to take me to the radiologist's office. So I enlisted the help of another friend, Kim. She picked me up; because I could not drive in the mental state I was in. I am not a big proponent of Valium, but believe me, if I had had some on hand, I would have taken some. I could not stop my mind from racing. I thought I was headed for a stroke and was never going to be the same. It was truly a frightening day. Even as I write this, my arm is feeling funny and tears are in my eyes thinking back to it.

I went to the radiologist's office (the same office where my cancer had been found), and they led me to the ultrasound room, where they located a blood clot near my port. I was so scared that this blood clot would travel to my brain and I would no longer be the same person. But it didn't. The hematologist's office called me back four hours later after they got my results to tell me I was not in any medical danger, but they did tell me to come in on Monday.

I went to the office still a little spooked. The doctor told me the clot was a side effect of the port placement. The hematologist gave me two injections in my belly. This medicine helped to thin my blood. Then he gave me a thirty-day supply of syringes so I could inject myself. I needed to give myself a daily shot for as long as I had the port in my body. I continued for six weeks even after I got the port taken out.

The medication helped the swelling in my arm gradually decrease; after the first shot my arm felt less stiff. Within a few days, it felt physically better, but it took a few weeks for it to fully return to normal.

Now, if I hadn't been so scared that I was going to have a stroke, the thought of giving myself this shot daily would have put me over the edge. But I was relieved. As much as the whole blood clot scare put the fear of death in me, I was glad the daily shots were something that was very doable and made sense to me. My doctor explained that he could put me on an oral blood thinner or I could take the daily shots. He said the oral meds stayed in your body a lot longer than the shots, and came with many side effects. So although the idea of giving myself a shot in the stomach every day was something I never thought I could do, it was better than the oral meds.

In the beginning, Frank gave me the shots. I knew it was something I could do if I needed to, but I was trying to lessen the amount of stress in my life. I really looked at it as something he did lovingly for me on a daily basis. After he gave me my shot, I would say, "Thanks for saving my life today!"

Eventually, after four months, I got up the courage to give myself the shots. The needle came with the medicine already loaded. All I needed to do was inject myself. I cleaned my belly with an alcohol pad and stuck the needle through my skin, which was really a strange feeling. But I couldn't push the plunger part down. I sat there with the needle stuck in my belly without being able to push the medication into my body. I pulled it out and asked Frank to inject me again. I successfully attempted it again a few days later. This time I committed to sticking myself and pushing the medication into my body, and somehow it worked. From that day on, I injected myself. I am still very proud of getting the courage to inject myself.

When I arrived at the office to get my next IPT, Marybeth questioned whether or not it was safe for me to use the port to receive my treatment. I told them the hematologist had given me permission. They called the hematologist's office, but it wasn't open yet. Frank and I sat in the IPT waiting room while various phone calls were made on my behalf. I decided as these calls were going on that I was not going to get my IPT that day. After discussing the situation with Frank, I was still stressed out from the blood clot episode, and now I was upset that the nurses thought it could pose a problem with my port. We decided it was best for me to skip treatment that week and go home and rest.

During that week off I was able to regroup and. I was unsure what "the universe" was trying to tell me. Was it trying to intervene here? I stopped and took notice of what was going on with my body and the circumstances around me. Was I not supposed to receive the IPT? I just wasn't sure, so I did nothing. When I say nothing, I mean I put my IPT treatments on hold. I gave myself time to pray, meditate, and eat good, healthy food. I quieted and cleared my mind, and then waited to "get my answer" about what to do next. By the end of the week, I felt 100 percent. I knew what I was doing was best for me. My arm felt better, the medical clearance was all straightened out, and I was in a better frame of mind to get on with treatments. I was now mentally and physically ready to forge ahead.

The rest of the IPT sessions went without a hitch. Sometimes Frank, my sister-in-law, or a friend would keep me company during my five-hour treatment, but I enjoyed going by myself too. I know that sounds strange, but it was an opportunity to be strong. Obviously, if I was physically or mentally not able to do it by myself, I would get the help. It felt good to be capable of driving myself to and from the appointments. I relished the quiet time. During the hour-long drive, I would listen to the comedy channel and try to laugh the whole time. On the way home, I would listen to music that I could sing along with and sing at the top of my lungs. I enjoyed watching funny TV shows or movies on my iPad during treatment. It was my way of "checking out" to what was going on around me with something funny. The nurses would get the biggest kick out of me laughing by myself.

Massage

Dr. Linchitz's office was not your typical cancer treatment facility. The office offers yoga and massage for both caretakers and patients. I took them up on the massage many times. I really enjoyed having the massages during treatment. It was a way of allowing my body to relax. Plus, it was nice for my body to receive "good" messages while under the stress of cancer.

I took this idea one step further and went regularly for massages throughout the course of my treatment. Massage was definitely something filed under self-care. I know it may sound indulgent to get massages once or even twice a week. I kept telling myself, *You only get cancer once, so why not?*

Studies show that massage improves immune function and releases endorphins that act as natural painkillers. Massage even lessens depression and anxiety. I always felt better emotionally and physically after a massage. My mind always seemed clearer. I had more sense of clarity and calmness, which was something I definitely needed during this difficult time.

David Servan-Schreiber writes about the effect of massage on the body in his book *Anticancer*. "Research at the University of Miami has shown that three weekly thirty-minute massages slowed down the production of stress hormones and increased the number of Natural Killer cells (also known as NK cells) in women with breast cancer," he writes.

The massages felt like an opportunity for something nice to happen to my body. At the various doctor visits, touch became stress producing. Even though the office staff was "nice" during my chemo treatments, the whole experience was still very stressful. Massage allowed me to relax back into my body and give it some much-deserved love.

During IPT, my life was consumed with cancer treatments. The nurses at treatment became my good friends, since I was there sometimes twice a week for five to six hours at a time. I was either going to treatment or resting my body for the next treatment. I was committed to doing nothing but staying healthy. I had the opportunity not to work during my cancer treatment, so staying healthy became my work. I had my massages, experimented with food, researched various cancer diets, committed to detoxifying my body with hot yoga, and continued to exercise moderately. I did feel healthy during my treatments, and I think that's something we can all strive for.

END OF IPT

Fourteen sessions of IPT flew by, and thank goodness most of them went off without a hitch. The only reoccurring problem was accessing the port. During my last treatment session, I wanted to express my gratitude for the staff. I brought in a basket of Edible Arrangements fruit for them to share. I went by myself for my last treatment. Frank offered to come with me, but I felt like this was something I wanted to do on my own. I left the office with tears of joy streaming down my face. I was so relieved to put that part of cancer treatment behind me. I had confronted and gone through the unthinkable. As I drove home by myself with my sunroof open and the music blaring, a special song came on the radio: Steve Winwood's "Back in the High Life Again." I sang every word at the top of my lungs.

> It used to seem to me
> That my life ran on too fast
> And I had to take it slowly
> Just to make the good parts last

That song spoke to me years ago when it was popular, and again as I completed my treatment. It felt like I was back in the high life again! That song became the theme of the evening as I celebrated with family and friends at our favorite restaurant.

How I Survived My IPT Treatments

1. **Rested.** I gave my body an opportunity to do what it needed to do: heal and rest up from the drugs I was putting into my system.
2. **Continued to watch shows that made me laugh.** Studies have shown that laughing reduces pain, decreases stress-related hormones, and boosts your immune system.
3. **Cleared my schedule of any stressful events.** I wanted my life to be filled with simple things while I was undergoing treatment so I could focus on healing.
4. **Ate organic produce.** I put high-quality antioxidant foods into my body to help it stay healthy.
5. **Experimented with different ways of getting more greens into my diet (see chapter 7 for details).** I started making smoothies and juices to add more green vegetables on a daily basis.
6. **Started really focusing on the present moment.** I consciously focused on the here and now, and tried not to worry about the future.
7. **Found a therapist.** I found a professional who could help me deal with my cancer diagnosis.

Part 3: Burn—Radiation

I gave myself time between treatments to relax and spend time with my family. That's right—I took two months off from cancer. It's one of the best benefits of being CEO. I finished chemo treatments the last week of June and took "off from cancer" for July and August. I didn't visit any doctors, except in late August to have my port removed. I probably would not have been in such a rush to have that done, but I was still giving myself daily injections of a blood thinner.

I relaxed with my family for the months of July and August. I enjoyed all that summer has to offer here on Long Island. All three of my kids sail in the summer, so dropping them off at class forced me to go down to the water and take in the beautiful views and calmness. The summer was the perfect opportunity to really relax, swim, eat locally grown, organic foods, and tend to my garden. I was so happy to have the most difficult part of my cancer treatment behind me.

Since the IPT treatments were finished, the port was no longer necessary. It was time to get it out! I made the appointment with Dr. McCloy to have the port removed in late August. Because this was surgery number three, I knew what to expect at the hospital, which antinausea meds worked best for me, and which pain medications I had adverse reactions to. I was more in control. I had the port removed in the morning, and the next day I attended a sailing awards ceremony for the kids. I still needed to give myself the shots to thin my blood for six more weeks, but there was an end in sight.

I remember the last day I had to give myself the injection. My belly was full of bruises and bloated from six months' worth of puncture wounds. I relished that last injection. I felt gratitude for what that blood thinner drug did for me, and I enjoyed closing yet another chapter of my cancer story.

How I Kept My Immunity Up

During my time off from cancer treatments, I still took cancer seriously. I wanted to keep my immune system up and functioning at full capacity, so I took my diet up a notch. Since it was summer, eating local, organic green vegetables was easy. I took full advantage of everything my garden, friends' gardens, and farmers' markets had to offer. My breakfasts were filled with fresh, local, organic, in-season fruit served over steel-cut oats. My lunch comprised various green salads filled with nuts and homemade dressings. Dinner included whatever vegetables were ready for picking in the garden or bought from the farm stand. I became the master of grilling vegetables such as zucchini, carrots, onions, and garlic. I would make enough to eat for dinner that night and then make a wrap for lunch the next day with leftovers. I experimented with what tasted good, gave me energy, and was easy to prepare. My diet consisted mostly of vegetables, beans, and occasionally some local, organic meats.

While I gave my body the opportunity to rest and repair itself, I fed it with supplements as well as foods. I took herbs that Dr. Linchitz recommended such as ginseng, curcumin, and astragalus to help build up my immunity before I started radiation.

By September, my vacation from cancer treatment was over and it was time to start the voyage of radiation. Radiation is not nearly as controversial as other cancer treatments. Study after study shows that radiation reduces the risk of cancer recurrence, especially breast cancer. Again, I talked with various types of doctors about their opinion of radiation and even the most "alternative" doctors recommended it. I was fully committed to doing the radiation, knowing that if I hated it or had bad side effects, I would reevaluate my situation.

Here is how Professor Martha C. Monroe and Dr. Barbara F. Shea describe radiation in the breast cancer series on the University of Florida IFAS extension website:

> Radiation treatments for cancer come from machines powered by electricity. A linear accelerator releases photons (packets of light energy) and electrons (negatively charged subatomic particles) in a concentrated and carefully aimed pattern designed to target cancer cells. By using a small dose repeatedly every day over several weeks, radiation treatment helps kill cancer cells.
>
> The radiation treatment works by bombarding cells with energy that breaks apart molecules. This generates electrons (one type of free radical) that spin off to hit other cells and disrupt

DNA synthesis. Both healthy and cancer cells are damaged during this treatment. The daily dose of radiation is kept low enough to allow healthy tissues to regenerate.

I was given the name of a radiologist from my oncologist. The course of radiation treatment for breast cancer is pretty straightforward. I interviewed one radiation oncologist, as my expectations were quite different when it came to radiation treatment. I just wanted to keep my head down and do what I needed to do. The doctor was fine, he listened to my questions, he explained things adequately, and best of all, the location was near my house. Location was very important, because I would drive there five days a week for the next six and a half weeks. Yes, that's thirty-three treatments. I wanted my treatments to take place in an office setting rather than a hospital setting. I wanted my treatments to go as quickly and easily as possible.

Before I could even start the radiation treatments, several prep appointments needed to take place. By this point in my cancer treatment, I was ready for just about anything. But the next step seemed to push me over the edge; it was the tattoo session. Yes, I was upset about having to get a tattoo on my body to mark where I would be zapped with radiation. Yes, I am a big baby! My friends thought I was joking about it. They could not believe that after all I'd been through, the tattoo had me so upset. I was scared it was going to hurt as well as upset that there would be another physical reminder of my cancer.

Tattoos are used in radiation therapy so the radiation therapist can precisely pinpoint the area needing treatment. The permanent markings are crucial for ensuring the accurate targeting of the tumor area. It allows the technician to line up the treatment fields more quickly, making each treatment session run more smoothly.

Even before I went in for tattoos, I called the office and asked what the technician's favorite treat was. They told me Brian loved candy. Although it goes against my idea of spreading health, I decided to put together a bag of high-quality chocolate as a gift for him. When the day came for me to get my tattoos, I let the radiation therapist know I was scared. Brian (a.k.a. my new best friend once I showed him the bag of treats waiting for him after the session) put me at ease, explaining that the needle would go just below the skin, not down to the breastbone as I had imagined. He showed me that the tattoo size would be equivalent to that of a pin and that I would have only two markings. He told me he would talk me through every part of the procedure so I would be aware of what was going on.

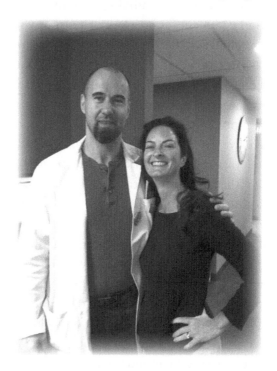

Brian, the guy who gave me my first tattoo.

He took many measurements while I was lying on the MRI table. I could handle that part. I had learned to use it as an opportunity to tune out and practice my abdominal breathing. After about thirty minutes of measurements, Brian let me know it was tattoo time. Instead of being all worked up about it, I gave in. I said, "Okay, do what you need to do."

And guess what? It wasn't bad at all. The needle didn't hurt. It was small, and he didn't need to go deep into my skin. The tattoos were small, and only one is visible to me, and only if I look really closely. With that part behind me, I was ready to commit to going through radiation.

I really didn't know what to expect when it came to radiation other than it shouldn't hurt and I might be tired. Oh yeah, and the doctor told me to expect a burn.

When I pulled up for my first of thirty-three radiation appointments, I sat in the car by myself, hesitant to start this next part of my cancer treatment. I wanted to gather my thoughts and be emotionally strong as I entered the building. I turned on the radio, and again, the universe "spoke" to me through song. Yet another Talking Heads song came on, called "This Must Be the Place."

Tears proceeded to stream down my face while I listened to the words:

> Home is where I want to be
> Pick me up and turn me around
> I feel numb—burn with a weak heart
> (so I) guess I must be having fun

I laughed out loud while listening to this confirmation that this was where I needed to be. I sat and listened to the song, and it changed my perspective. I went from fearful to empowered. I knew deep down that "This Must Be the Place." I got out of the car, marched inside, and signed my name on the radiation patient sign-in sheet.

I made fast friends with Judy, the receptionist at the radiation office. She made me feel welcomed, and I knew she would keep a watchful eye on me if I needed it, and I did. There was a day when the waiting room was overfilled with patients. She brought me to the back so we could talk during the long wait to get my treatment. Judy also kept me company when I needed to do blood work.

Treatment day one and treatment day thirty-three were all the same to me. I put on a hospital gown that opened in the front, signed the "official" radiation room book, and walked through a steel door with the "Danger Radioactive" sign on it, which always made me chuckle. I would climb up on the exam table that looked like a MRI machine. The technician would open my gown on the left side and circle my incision scar with a black Sharpie marker and then line my tattoos up with the radiation machine. The technicians always recited the same two measurements once I was lined up, and then left the room. I would lie on the table motionless, waiting for my invisible radiation treatment to begin. It took about five minutes with the machine clicking and doing what it needed to do to keep me cancer-free. My eyes were shut and I focused on my breathing. My eyes remained shut during the whole five minutes of treatment, so I can't tell you in detail what was really going on with that machine. But I do remember that part of the machine would come in close to my body.

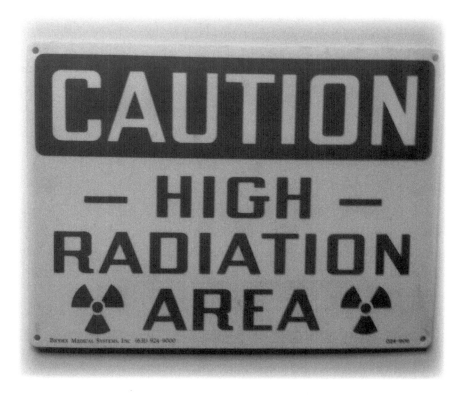

I would pass this sign everyday as I walked into the radiation treatment room.

Radiation was a completely different experience from the IPT treatment. With the IPT, you see the fluorescent yellow toxic drugs going into your body. A nurse has to administer the drugs, so there is physical contact with your cancer caretakers. The radiation itself is invisible. You are left with the physical remnants of what the radiation leaves behind with its burn, but the actual daily radiation is a very cold and sterile feeling. Now, don't get me wrong, the technicians were friendly and caring. But the whole thing about climbing up onto a cold examination table for this machine to shoot these invisible rays into my breast tissue was just an odd concept.

I suffered only minor side effects from radiation treatment, and I think it's because I took such good care of my body with my diet. I used natural lotions to help myself heal from the radiation burn. My doctor warned me that I would get a radiation burn during treatment, especially because I had such fair skin.

Let me explain something here. When the doctor said "burn," I envisioned a small round burn on the skin of my breast—something the size and shape of a penny. In my mind that was the size of the "radiation." Boy, was I wrong! About halfway through the thirty-three treatments, I started to see the burn in the mirror: a strange triangle shape, about six inches wide, starting below my collarbone and ending above my nipple. As I proceeded with the radiation treatments, only one small section of my breast was red, dry, and later appeared raw. It became quite obvious to me while I stared into the mirror where the radiation was zapping my body.

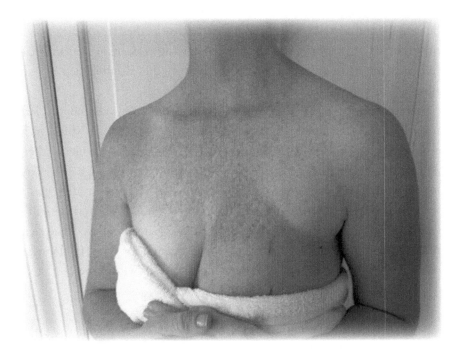

My radiated breast near the end of treatment.

I took special precautions with my skin immediately after treatment and before I went to bed at night. I used two products every day: Melaleuca's brand of skin lotion called Renew, and a lavender essential oil from Young Living Oils. I would bring a sample size of Renew into the changing room with me and rub it into the radiated section of my breast after treatment. I would use the high-grade lavender oil on my skin at night before bedtime.

Note: I recently had a dermatologist appointment six months post radiation. The dermatologist could not believe how great my radiated skin looked. She said it was the best radiated skin she had ever seen! She could not believe I had completed thirty-three radiation treatments. Amazing, right?

The radiation oncologist also warned me that I might feel fatigued during my six weeks of treatments. I stayed diligent with my clean, healthy eating, drinking my green smoothies, and resting when I needed to. I did not take any supplements during radiation. Several studies show it could be detrimental to treatment. Radiation therapy makes free radicals as a means of killing cancer cells, and the goal of antioxidants is to neutralize free radicals, so I opted to keep up the healthy diet. I continued to run (slowly) and take yoga classes during my treatments.

I created one big fun distraction during my radiation treatments. I left inspirational Sticky notes in the radiation changing room. I would pick a quote that meant something to me, write it in black Sharpie marker, and post it on the corner of the mirror. I posted a new message every day for thirty days. I never got to see the reaction of the person after me. I wanted to believe that my message brought a smile to the next patient's face. I envisioned my inspirational notes changing the intention of the next person hopping onto the examination table waiting for them in the next room. I loved coming up with quotes that resonated within me.

Here are some of my favorite notes:

- You are strong and healthy.
- Do your best and forget the rest.
- Every day may not be great, but there is something great in every day.
- Don't tell me the sky is the limit, because there are footprints on the moon.

- Whether you think you can or you can't, you're right.
- Don't look back—you're not going that way.
- May today bring you peace, tranquility, and harmony.

I finished radiation treatment right before Thanksgiving. Frank came with me to my last appointment. I wanted him to meet the people who had seen me on a daily basis for the last six and a half weeks. I also wanted Frank there because I had a "check-out" appointment with the radiation oncologist. I knew my blood pressure would be elevated for the appointment, because I was anxious. I think I was scared the doctor was going to tell me I wasn't finished. I needed Frank by my side to help me over my last hurdle. I wanted him to speak on my behalf if I couldn't get my thoughts together. I wanted him to say no to the doctor if he suggested that I have more treatments.

At that last appointment I was reminded yet again that I was not a typical patient. One of the things the doctor said was that I could resume my physical activity level. He said that many patients find that their energy level returns within a few weeks. I found that funny, because while I was undergoing my treatment, I participated in two 5K running races. My energy level was just fine. I knew that my lotions, healthy diet, rest, and continued exercise were helping me combat the side effects of radiation.

The doctor reminded me (without him knowing it, of course) that I was doing something right here. I never had to stop treatment because of either elevated or decreased white blood cell counts or because my immune system was compromised. I felt great for someone who had just been through a horrible, unthinkable event. Why was I okay? The body that I had been so upset with for giving me cancer was now reminding me that maybe because I took such good care of myself, I was thriving.

Two key components to keeping sane during my cancer adventure were giving my body the opportunity to rest and taking treatments at my own pace. I filled my body with great whole foods; I crowded out fearful thoughts with the help of therapy and stayed close with my family. With my exercise of yoga and running, I was able to keep my mind in the present. I made myself a top priority and rested when I needed to rest and didn't feel guilty about it.

I am finished with cancer treatment now. Every imaginable test has been done to my blood, urine, and saliva. When I went back for my first follow-up cancer testing, Dr. Linchitz told me that my tests revealed that I am the envy of a healthy person. Every lab test result indicates that I am perfectly healthy! Yay! To say I felt relieved would not do it justice. I shared with Dr. Linchitz my original intuition that cancer was not something I would ever get again. He agreed with me.

I really live by the idea that not one thing gave me cancer, and not one treatment cured my cancer. It was a compilation of events that both sparked it and cured it. The same goes for my after-cancer care. I don't believe one drug can keep me healthy or that food or exercise is enough. It's a combination of everything. It goes back to what I learned at my time at Integrative Nutrition, that it's not one thing that makes someone healthy; rather, it's a variety of things such as relationships, exercise, food, and spirituality.

WHAT KEPT ME SANE DURING THIRTY-THREE RADIATION TREATMENTS

1. **Stayed local:** I picked a local office to receive radiation treatments so I didn't have to travel far every day.
2. **Kept my head in the books:** I always brought a book or my phone to keep me busy while I waited.
3. **Hydrated:** I continued to drink half my weight in water each day.
4. **Got green:** I increased my intake of green veggies, along with fruits and berries.
5. **Treated my skin:** I committed to taking care of my radiated skin with a lotion without toxic parabens. (More on that in chapter 7.)
6. **Slept In:** I rested when I felt tired and gave my body a chance to heal from treatment.
7. **Motivated to move:** I actually ran two 5K races during my treatment. I found that exercise helped with depression and kept my energy levels elevated. But I never pushed it and exercised only when I had energy to.

8. **Focused on gratitude**: With my sticky notes, I made each treatment about something other than myself. It felt good to give back to others even with this small gesture.

Chapter 5

Sex, Drugs, and Fear

You would think that once I ended my cancer treatments, my life would return to mostly normal. Well, I soon found that I still had a lot to process. Three things weighed heavily on my mind after navigating my cancer maze. One of them was dealing with the emotional scars that cancer left behind. How could I reclaim my breast as part of my body and not think of it as a medical emergency? Another was deciding whether or not to take a drug (with some serious side effects) that had the potential to prevent my cancer from coming back. Last, how did I deal with all the fear of having cancer and wondering if it would come back?

Sex and My Breast

After the surgery, I had to change how I think of my breasts. It was hard to think of them as sexual again because they were clinical for so long. I had forgotten all the joy they had brought me! Besides sexually, they successfully fed three kids for the first year of their life. Although the physical scars are almost nonexistent—the surgery scar is faded, my radiated skin that was so badly burned is back to normal, and the tattoos are something I don't even tune in to very often—I am left with psychological scars. I consider myself lucky. I met women whose breasts were disfigured because of surgery as well as radiation. If I had trouble getting past my various "scars," I can only imagine how other women have dealt with this situation.

I will make this part brief because I know Frank will be mortified that I am sharing details of our sex life. My postsurgical feelings about my breasts were reminiscent of breast-feeding the babies. During my breast-feeding period, my breasts had a purpose—they were feeding an infant. Now my breasts took on a new meaning. My left breast has been touched in such a clinical way for a year that it will take some time to feel normal again. Touching my breast is not physically painful, but it's still awkward to have it caressed. My left breast looks fine and you would never know that it had had cancer removed from it. But on an emotional level, I am still healing.

I was recently introduced to Barbara Musser, author of *Sexy After Cancer*. She has dedicated her therapy practice to helping women and their partners deal with loving their bodies and themselves post cancer. In her book and at her seminars, she shares her own breast cancer story and gives practical tips and exercises to help women connect with their own radiant sexual energy. She lays the foundation for healing, accepting, forgiving, and loving their changed body. She offers helpful communication techniques for women to share with their partners about intimacy.

After reading her book, I realized I was not alone in how I felt about my breasts. I felt relieved just knowing that my feelings were not unusual. I understood that time wasn't the only thing that was going to heal my "scars." I needed to do some work on me and how I viewed my new body. I am currently doing her daily exercises that include looking at myself in the mirror and repeating healing statements. Musser says using the mirror as a healing tool is a powerful aid in coming to terms with yourself and making peace with your body. By doing exercises in the mirror, you are changing the structure inside your brain and creating new neural pathways. She goes on to explain that when you do her mirror work for thirty consecutive days, you are re-creating the unconscious thoughts in your head, turning them into thoughts of love and acceptance.

Just recently I was reminded that injuries leave emotional scars. My dog Zoe had an injured leg. The veterinarian told us that although her leg was healed on a physical level, she still might not climb the stairs, out of fear. Once she forgets she was ever injured, she will climb the stairs without even thinking. Wouldn't you know it took about four weeks for her to remember she was fine! She climbs the stairs just fine now. I just thought this was too funny. Zoe too has emotional scars that she needs to get over.

Drugs or No Drugs

Typically the next phase of breast cancer treatment includes the drug Tamoxifen. This synthetic hormone is a type of chemotherapy in pill form that blocks estrogen production, which is beneficial to women with estrogen-receptor positive cancer (which I had). Tamoxifen has been shown to inhibit the growth of cancer cells and in some cases prevent it.

So if this little pill can do so much, why wouldn't I take it? Well, it does have some serious side effects. One of them is blood clotting, and since I had the blood clot with the port, I didn't want to take any chances with this medication. My conservative oncologist was even hesitant about recommending it to me. The other major side effects from Tamoxifen are deep vein thrombosis, endometrial cancer, uterine cancer, stroke, hot flashes, and cataracts.

The other issue I have with this drug is that drug companies produce much of the research about it. When I read research studies, I look to see who funded the research. I look at who is actually being studied and who is being left out. A study done at the University of California, Davis, looked at the benefits of Tamoxifen on the life expectancy of women. The problem is that the women in the study had hysterectomies and were no longer at risk of developing uterine cancer. Did they leave out the women with a uterus on purpose to skew the data?

Still, the decision not to take the Tamoxifen was a difficult one. I talked with my oncologist Dr. V about it, along with various other medical doctors. Everyone had an opinion. I felt like it would have been easy to go in blindly and take their recommendations. The research can be a full-time job at times. Frank and I read many documents and talked with many doctors about it. I just felt as though there was a more natural way of treating my body.

I have decided not to take any meds at this point, but rather to investigate other, less toxic ways of addressing the extra estrogen that my body produces. I am working with two different doctors to be sure my estrogen levels stay within normal limits through lifestyle and dietary changes, including supplements. (Learn more in chapter 7.)

I also went back to my original gut feeling that I am healthy and strong, and that cancer is something that I will not revisit in my life. I reminded myself of my premise that not one thing gave me cancer so just one thing is not going to cure me. Was Tamoxifen the "one" thing that was going to keep cancer at bay? I'm not sure, but at this time it's not something I feel good about taking. I could not imagine taking a drug on a daily basis that I did not feel good about. In my case I think that would be more detrimental than the drug itself.

Deciding whether or not to take Tamoxifen was a big decision. Here's some of the thinking I used to decide whether or not to take a drug:

1. First I asked, "How long has the drug been on the market?"
2. I familiarized myself with the research studies done on the drug.
3. What is the drug supposed to accomplish?
4. What are the side effects? Are they short term or long term?
5. I asked my doctor, "How long will I need to be on it before I can see if it is working for me?"
6. If I don't like the way my body feels, can I get off it easily enough?
7. Are there any alternatives to the drug?
8. I sought out other types of doctors to get their opinion.

Dealing with Fear

As positive and healthy as I felt, fear still had a way of creeping into my head to say, "Boo!" I was scared of dying, scared that the cancer might come back, and scared that my body would never be the same once I completed treatment. So although I was feeling strong physically, I knew I needed more help to feel strong mentally.

I had a previous connection with hypnotherapy. I had worked with a hypnotherapist back in 2003 that helped me deal with the fear of getting seasick. For Frank's fortieth birthday we went on a tour of the Galapagos Islands, which meant we needed to be on a boat for seven days. The tour boat we were on was quite small for my standards and for sailing in the Pacific Ocean! I got more anxious instead of excited as the trip was approaching, and a therapist friend of mine recommended I see a hypnotherapist. She had seen firsthand the great results he had produced. I used hypnotherapy to help me relax so I could enjoy my trip to the

Galapagos Islands, and it worked! With the help of Dr. Bezmen, in just a few sessions I was able to lower my anxiety level by using various relaxation techniques. I was able to really enjoy our trip.

Once I was down to every other week for chemotherapy treatments, I made the time to talk with a therapist. Since I knew he had helped me with my mind-body connection before, I decided to try him again. William Bezmen, PhD, completed a fellowship in clinical hypnotherapy and is a clinical specialist in psychiatric nursing. He's had a private practice since 1980 and teaches classes in hypnosis as well.

Dr. Bezmen guided me into healing my body from the inside out. He helped me come up with a healing journey that I could take myself on each day. This type of therapy is based on the theory that cells carry memories, and I really liked that idea. I wanted to release those "phantom memories" that were stored in my cells. With my therapist's help, I worked on releasing any limiting thoughts that didn't serve me so that when the new cells reproduced, they got the message to reproduce healthy cells. Sounds similar to how chemotherapy works, just on a whole other level. Pretty cool, right?

My intent was to put new thoughts into my body. I gained an understanding that the fears would still be there; I just learned how to hear them and then release them *before they settled into my body.* I focused on filling my head with healing thoughts. It's the same theory as with food. I was crowding out the "fearful" thoughts (processed foods) with more positive thoughts (higher-quality foods).

Dr. Bezmen made a fifteen-minute recording specifically for me to listen to each day. My CD takes me on a healing journey through nature with relaxation exercises and visualizations to help still my body and mind. My journey takes me through the woods en route to a Native American village where a fire ceremony is waiting for me. I stand at the fire, letting all my fears or limiting thoughts enter my mind, and then I energetically release the fearful thoughts into an imaginary white birch log and place the log on the fire. I stand there watching my fears being released into the air. When I complete my imaginary walk through the woods, I feel refreshed and clear headed.

I still see Dr. Bezmen twice a month. Frank reminds me how powerful my thoughts can be and that this is the most important part of my cancer treatment. We have a quote from Henry Ford hanging in our house: "Whether you think you can or you can't, you're right." Seeing that sign on a daily basis reminds me that I have the power to stay healthy and strong.

Some days, especially when my body and mind feel out of balance, the fear strikes. I try not to let it take me to a depressed, nongrounded place. I really try to meditate on being healthy and strong. I cling to that feeling that every cell of my body is healed and I am a healthy, vibrant, happy person.

When fear takes over, I know it's time to stop what I'm doing and reevaluate my schedule. I usually start looking at the number of activities I have said yes to and decide whether each one is bringing me stress or helping me stay healthy. Another activity that helps me stay grounded is cooking homemade, healthy meals. I am sure to enlist my three kids to help with the prep work, so we all spend some time together.

I also turn to yoga when I feel out of balance and stressed. I've kept this practice going on and off for more than twenty years. It wasn't until I got a diagnosis of cancer that I really reaped the benefits of practicing yoga on and off the mat. I learned (after hearing it for years) about doing a pose and then leaving it—truly understanding what it means to do it and then let it go. I practiced staying in the moment, not thinking about the last pose, or the next pose, but staying grounded in what I was doing at that moment. I know all that sounds really out there, but having an instructor remind me to let go over and over again helped.

Yoga also gave me the opportunity to quiet my mind and body; something I really needed after I felt like my body had let me down. Yoga literally forced me to look in the mirror at my body and show it gratitude for what it was capable of doing. At the end of every yoga class, the instructor would close with a meditation. The meditation lasted between five and ten minutes and was an opportunity to release negative thoughts and replace them with energizing, healing thoughts. Yoga became something that I really looked forward to doing. I could work on releasing tension in my injured arm, detoxing my body, and making my mind stronger.

The other thing I try to remember is that not every pain means cancer. The first time I had an ache in my armpit, I found it difficult to keep from automatically thinking cancer. I've learned to literally stop the story in my head, which is completely blown out of proportion, and remind myself that I am healthy. I remember that I was checked just a few months ago and will be checked again in a few more months. I remember all the great test results I have gotten. Sometimes I can get fear out of my head by reminding myself that the future is promised to no one. I tell myself that I could die in a car accident just as easily as anyone else.

Fear is a crummy four-letter word that I still deal with. I try not to let it cripple me or take over my head. That's why the yoga, meditation, and therapy are so important to me. All three modalities remind me to stay grounded in the present and to let go of those thoughts that don't serve me, and help me bring in the good, energizing, healing thoughts that are useful for my body.

MY FEAR-BUSTING TOOLS:

- Therapy
- Meditation
- Reducing daily stress
- Yoga

Chapter 6

Things You Have to Deal With When You Have Cancer, a.k.a. the Crappy Parts of Cancer

AGAIN, I TURNED TO MUSIC to help me deal with what was going on around me. The song "Where Are You Going?" by the Dave Matthews Band came to mind when I was dealing with what I call the crappy parts of cancer. I just wanted to tell people I have no idea where I'm going. I am no superman (or superwoman). I'm just looking for answers. I'm just doing what I need to do for me.

> I am no Superman
> I have no reasons for you
> I am no hero
> Oh, that's for sure

THE JOURNEY

The strange thing about cancer is the journey. Before I had cancer, I read and heard people talk about this "cancer journey." When you hear that word *journey,* it sounds fun. Cancer is anything but fun. The journey involves many people. When I started, I thought Frank and I would go through it together, but I soon realized there were many others who took the journey with me. Besides my immediate family members, many friends came along and showed up in amazing ways.

Friends came to doctor visits with me when Frank was working. Friends drove my kids places. Friends helped with food when I was too tired to cook. Friends called just to cheer me up. Other friends just sent me good thoughts. I never thought of myself as a belonging to a larger group of women, but I realized I did belong. I had this whole network of people to help me on every level. Some people helped on a daily basis, some weekly, and others whenever. I never experienced a time while I was undergoing treatment when there wasn't a friend available for me.

I realized how important friends were and wasn't surprised when I read in the Nurses' Health Study that if a woman with breast cancer could name ten friends, she had a four times better chance of surviving her illness than women who could not. The study also said that the geographical proximity of these friendships was not significant.

MAKING A COMMUNICATIONS PLAN FOR CANCER

When I got my diagnosis of cancer, I told Frank and the kids at the same time. It never occurred to me not to tell my kids. I was unsure what it meant to have cancer, but I knew it was something way too big to keep from them. Since they didn't go outside the home for school, they didn't have to explain to the kids at school or a random mother who might approach them. The day I had my lumpectomy, I left before they were up in the morning and was home by the afternoon. As for the cancer treatments, they never saw any side effects. I never lost my hair from the chemo treatment, and they never saw the burn from the radiation. They saw me as this healthy mom who just rested a lot, and they knew to be extra nice to me. Because they are individuals, it probably affected them each differently and will probably continue to affect their lives as it does mine.

Telling my extended family members about cancer went fine. But telling them which treatments I decided to do was uncomfortable. You would think by now after the home-birth and homeschooling decisions, the idea of not doing mainstream cancer treatments would not come as a surprise, but it did. Everyone had an opinion. I dealt with this by letting Frank handle those conversations. Thankfully, he had some credibility with them since he's a doctor.

I found it difficult to let friends know I had cancer. It's a sticky topic. I told my closest friends by calling them on the phone. I kept them updated on my progress and treatment through texts and e-mails. I asked people in different parts of my life to help spread the word. I trusted them not to gossip about it, but I knew they would tell people who needed to know. I found it helpful to have a spokesperson. I would let a few friends know what was going on, and then they in turn would tell others. A few friends composed e-mails on my behalf that I never read, but I'm glad they found a way to let people know.

I didn't mind people knowing that I had cancer; I just didn't want to be the one to tell them. But let's be clear about friends. I have lived in my community since 1996 so I know a lot of people. I run into people around town all the time. And I felt uncomfortable telling someone I ran into at the supermarket about this personal health crisis. It felt awkward to tell them I had cancer, so I didn't. If I ran into people in town who knew me but didn't know about the cancer, I didn't tell them. Simple.

I also didn't have the energy or desire to retell my cancer story over and over, so I turned to social media. On Facebook, I felt free to post updates for whoever wanted to read them. My network was still small at the time. My Facebook friends kept me company while I waited at doctors' offices, and I found it a nice distraction. I started a blog for extended family and close friends to read about details of my treatment. It helped me keep an account of my experience along the way.

I can only imagine how it was for Frank at work. Patients routinely ask, "How's Christine?" And he decided to answer, "She's great." He never knew for sure if they knew about my cancer or if they were just being polite. He let his office staff know about my diagnosis in a meeting, and then it became an unwritten policy that people didn't talk about it. His office was a place for him to escape cancer and focus on his patients and recharge for me.

I am still ambivalent about letting people know I had cancer because of the simple fact that I am still affected by their responses. I don't want to hear about their family member, friend, or coworker who just died of cancer. Unfortunately, I've heard that way too much. Those stories still rock me to the core. Some people even go into detail and tell horror stories. I try to nip those stories in the bud by saying, "If the story is sad, I don't want to hear it." The last thing I want to do is have these sad, scary stories in my head.

Once I let people know about my cancer, it felt like I was opening up a world of answering their questions. Do I look like a cancer expert?! I was also careful about divulging the kind of treatment I was doing because I didn't want to feel like I had to defend myself. People wanted to know about my surgery and whether I had my breast removed. Did I have them both removed? Why or why not? How was chemo? Was my breast tissue black from radiation? You would be surprised at the questions people ask. Sometimes I would answer them and sometimes I wouldn't. This was where I wanted to repeat the Dave Matthews lyrics:

> I am no Superman
> I have no reasons for you
> I am no hero
> Oh, that's for sure

To minimize my exposure to awkward moments, I took a break from a lot of social obligations. I valued my "me" time and spent much of my time resting and recuperating. I was practicing the ultimate self-care by letting go of my responsibilities. Frank and the kids took over my mommy duties, and I didn't worry if I missed birthday parties, social events, or other activities that I would have felt compelled to attend before. "Fitting out" of the social scene allowed me time to heal.

On one of the few occasions when I did go to a party, I got blindsided when a Facebook friend approached me in a group and proceeded to ask me about my cancer. It was one of those moments when my heart sank and I didn't know if it was obvious that I was uncomfortable. Instead of acting upset, I smiled and said I was doing great and thanked him for checking in with me. I think I was so thrown because the question came out of left field. I had no idea he was actually reading my Facebook posts! I still wonder when I run into a friend and they ask how it's going whether they know about my cancer. I usually answer "Just great" and leave it at that.

My point in sharing these stories is that you have to decide what works best for you. I decided to honor what I was feeling and not worry about what others thought. Ultimately I needed all my emotional strength to keep me sane, so I chose not to worry about others' reactions. Plus, I chose to focus on talking about wellness, not sickness.

But here's a positive note that I want to share: I recently ran into three friends on three separate occasions. After I told them I was writing this book, all three said they had forgotten I had cancer. They each apologized for saying so, but they see me as this healthy, vibrant person, not as someone who had cancer. I love *those* kinds of stories.

THE HAIR THING

So it's time to talk about the whole hair thing. As you know, most people who do chemo lose their hair. When I was going through treatment, I would run into people who thought my real hair was a wig. Then came the question, why hadn't I lost my hair? Was this my opportunity to tell people I was not doing a mainstream cancer treatment? That there are other options? Most of the time I would just explain that I was doing a low dose chemotherapy treatment and leave it at that. The dosage of chemotherapy drug was so low that my hair did not fall out. Actually, it was quite the opposite. Because of the high dosage of vitamin C, my hair and nails were long and healthy. As I write, my hair is the longest it's ever been. I tell people, "Since I got to keep it during my ordeal with cancer, I'm growing it long for a while."

LYMPHEDEMA

One of the side effects of having lymph nodes removed can be lymphedema. Lymphedema is a condition where the fluid builds up in the tissue and causes swelling, usually in the arm or leg. After surgery, my oncologist referred me to the lymphedema center at the local hospital to familiarize myself with the signs and symptoms of developing this disease. I made an appointment at the center. They took measurements of the circumference of my arm from the fingertips to my armpit. I asked the lymphedema therapist about prevention, and she said there is not much literature on how to prevent it. I was pretty frustrated by the fact that no major studies had been done on prevention. The literature the clinic gave me was all about what I should do if I see swelling develop in my fingers and arm. One tip the lymphedema therapist suggested was getting a compression sleeve for flying. I know my hands and feet normally swell when I fly, so I thought this was something I wanted to get.

I was referred to a store that caters to woman with breast cancer for the compression sleeves. Along with the sleeves, the store carries special bras, wigs, and shirts with built-in bras. I was glad that I did not go to the store at the beginning of my journey; I would have cried just walking in. I had an airplane trip planned at the end of August, so I wanted to get these compression sleeves to prevent my chances of getting lymphedema. Besides getting the sleeves, the store owner helped me get refitted for new bras since my breasts had changed. I figured I would get new bras after the cancer treatment was all finished, because then my breasts would settle into their new shapes. It never occurred to me to get some during treatment.

It sounds so silly to think I would just wait until this ordeal was over to get a properly fitting bra! Besides fitting me for a bra she also suggested I purchase "bra filler" for the right side to help even out my breasts. These bras have a pocket sewn into the underside of the cup so that flesh-colored chicken cutlet–looking filler can be slipped into it. Now my breasts look like they're the same size again. Who would have thought the filler would be for the nonsurgical breast? According to my surgeon, it is not uncommon to have the affected breast be larger because of scar tissue from the surgery. To this day I wear my "special" bra with my chicken-cutlet filler!

THE PINKING OF MY CANCER JOURNEY

Cancer reminders are everywhere. I still get tons of postcards and phone call reminders from all the various cancer doctors for follow-up. TV, print ads, and news stories are always talking about it.

Then came my first Breast Cancer Awareness month. It was not easy navigating this month of raising consciousness while undergoing breast cancer treatment. I was writing about my radiation treatment on my blog in October at my local Panera Bread when one of the female workers approached me. She asked if I wanted to purchase a pink bagel to help cure cancer.

As I sat frozen in my chair writing about cancer, this worker unknowingly caught me totally off guard. I had to get this straight: a worker was walking around selling pink bagels for the Susan G. Komen Foundation on "my" behalf. Panera wanted me to spend one dollar on this pink bagel wrapped in plastic. Where do I begin to talk about all the things wrong with that? First of all, my stomach was sick just thinking of the woman going around the store collecting money for this horrible disease that I had. I had such a love-hate relationship with what was transpiring around me. I loved the fact that people wanted to help, but also hated the fact that people were nonchalantly donating money to "finding a cure." Was the "cure" a pink-dyed, white-flour, sugar-laden bagel wrapped in carcinogenic plastic? It didn't feel like finding a cure to me. It sounded like exploiting a disease.

Here I was trying to eat my greens three times a day and this woman was putting this pink bagel in the name of cancer in my face. It just didn't jive with me. The last thing I wanted to put in my body was a bagel, never mind it being pink! I felt pressured to buy this bagel in solidarity for breast cancer. Believe it or not, I reached into my wallet and found a dollar. The bagel sat in the plastic wrapper for weeks on my counter before I even remembered it was there. I had to remove myself from the mainstream belief that this bagel was going to help cure cancer. Even before I got my diagnosis, I had always had a problem with any group that glamorized a disease. The pink ribbon symbol didn't cut it. The whole idea that breast cancer is this pretty sisterhood disease is just not true.

Dozens of companies raise funds in the name of breast cancer. But how can they promote finding a cure while pushing products that have strong links to causing it? Examples include facial creams with a "breast cancer company" stamp on them that contain parabens, a known carcinogen, or various perfumes that have toxic chemicals in their ingredients.

And then there's the food companies cashing in too. Yoplait yogurt sold pink-lidded yogurt to raise money for breast cancer. Unfortunately, the yogurt came from cows stimulated by the artificial hormone rBGH, which studies have demonstrated increase the risk of breast cancer, according to the group PR Watch. KFC also jumped on the pink-washing bandwagon, selling pink buckets of fried chicken to help "end breast cancer forever." In the "Buckets for the Cure" campaign, you could buy a five-dollar bucket of fried food and KFC promised to donate fifty cents to fight breast cancer. I'm not even going to address the animal cruelty behind KFC; many websites are dedicated to exposing the horrifying details of how KFC suppliers treat their chickens. The issue I have is the potential cancer-causing ingredients in KFC's food.

The big problem I have with the Susan G. Komen Foundation is that they receive more than $55 million in annual revenue from corporate sponsors like Coca-Cola, General Mills, and KFC. These are not exactly health-minded groups that I would associate with. I don't think you need to be a healthy person to see that there is a problem with a company that claims to "Find a Cure" and associates themselves with a fast food company.

The heartbreaking truth is that not one dollar of these "Find a Cure" efforts is put toward prevention. No funds are going to boost awareness about the important role of vitamin D in fighting cancer, how sugar adds to cancer growth, or the beneficial effects mushrooms have against cancer. That truth makes me sad. Cancer is a billion-dollar business, and no one is looking to cure it, just treat it with drugs.

What About "Snake Oils"?

People bombarded me with alternative options throughout my cancer experience. Friends would tell me about arsenic cures, red wine remedies, colonics, coffee enemas, and other outside-the-box modalities. Although I appreciated my friends' gestures, it was up to me to decide which ones I wanted to investigate further.

More than one friend referred me to a guy who makes a powder for a shake. I was told he had great results with cancer and other diseases. I added him to my list of things to investigate, but I didn't do it right away.

I made time to check his organization out shortly after I committed to doing low-dose chemotherapy. His "group" offers support meetings once a month. Frank was not interested in going with me, so I asked my brother to come along. My brother has been around the block a few times, and I knew he would be open-minded about what this group was offering.

When we arrived at the meeting, we were greeted with hugs and welcomed to the group. The people who work for this organization were very nice but did not radiate a vision of health. In fact, most of them just didn't look healthy.

They also bashed other alternative treatments. Now, I really hate when one group of alternative treatments trashes another. They are all supposed to be in the same boat; don't they know? They also said their ideal client rejects traditional forms of treatment like chemo and radiation, which was hard for me as someone who believes in researching all the options.

But I stuck it out. After listening to their other clients who have tried the shake talk about their results, I was amazed. One person had stage 4 colon cancer and is now cancer-free after using this product. Another woman who had stage 3 liver cancer spoke about how she is also now cancer-free thanks to the shakes. A few more people spoke about the great results they saw after using this shake.

The man who developed this product had cancer himself and spoke about his own frustration with doctors not getting to the root cause of his illness. The medical community could treat him, but not cure him. So he took it upon himself to figure out how to fix his cancer with minerals and vitamins that were missing from his body. The shake contains many minerals along with proprietary ingredients.

My brother and I left the meeting wondering, "What did we just walk in on?" We felt like we had been in a time warp. The meeting had a strange vibe and was a little too "Kumbaya" for us. I've never been to an AA meeting, but I imagine this event could be similar. The idea that this shake had helped so many people did intrigue me. It was something I put in the back of my mind, but I was not ready to commit to drinking the shake three times a day and taking twelve cod-liver oil pills per day. I stayed in touch with this group via Facebook, continuing to read testimonials from people who swore by the product.

Once all my cancer treatments were complete, I decided to revisit the group. Again, I asked my brother to join me. Together we went with the intention to buy the shake. We were welcomed back, but we had to sit through another meeting, and I was required to tell my story before I could make a purchase. I kept my mouth shut when the people started putting down my IPT and radiation, saying how toxic they were for my body. (Sorry—at this point it was a done deal!)

We listened to how the shake would give my body what it needed to stay cancer-free. It would rebalance my body with the minerals it was missing and solve the "why" I got sick in the first place. Now, this whole idea really appealed to me. I agreed with treating the cause of the disease instead of just the disease. I bought my two containers of shake powder, which would last me through the month. Each one cost thirty dollars. I listened intently to the best ways to make the shake, what to mix it with, and when to take it.

Remember, my brother came with me for moral support and not with the intent to purchase. At one point he turned to me and said, "If this stuff does half the stuff it's supposed to do, I would make an infomercial for this guy." Then he proceeded to buy a month's supply for himself.

I decided to use the product for the next six months and reevaluate. I tried drinking the shake for the first week but had bad stomach pains. I called the organization and told them my symptoms, and they said I was the first person out of thousands to ever call with that complaint. I was a little annoyed that they didn't answer my question. I was still CEO and needed more information.

Without a satisfactory answer, I decided to half the dose. I took half the scoop with apple cider. It's important that if you are going to commit to doing things on a daily basis, you have to really enjoy them to make them work. I did not enjoy taking this product. I am pretty good at taking things that don't taste so great, but I really did not enjoy drinking this at all. I so wanted to add it to my cancer-fighting arsenal, and I really wanted to like it.

The jury is still out. I haven't given up on it completely; perhaps I will pull it out of the cabinet and try it again sometime soon. Maybe I will read something on their Facebook page that will remind me that I should try it again. But for now, it's not something that I am doing on a regular basis.

As for my brother (who was taking it for his type 1 diabetes), he stopped when he ran out of product.

I'm not adverse to remedies that seem out there. Just because this one didn't work for me doesn't mean I stopped alternative treatments all together. I continue to research and keep an eye out for things that could work for me.

Chapter 7

My Simple and Doable Stay-Healthy Guide

Now that I've taken you through my cancer journey, I would like to share some of my daily practices to remain cancer-free. Just as it was important for me to take an active role in my treatment, it's been important for me to feel active and empowered about my future health. Many parts of my life look different now. I've developed tools to help me feel healthy and strong. Sometimes I use a few of my tools, and other times I use everything I've got. When I start to feel stressed or out of balance, I know I need to stop and remember what's in my toolbox.

It never occurred to me that cancer could actually come back. I know that sounds silly, but it was something that I hadn't thought of until I read Dr. David Servan-Schreiber's book *Anticancer*, where he mentions his cancer coming back. I remember lying in bed reading and thinking, did I just read this right? He had cancer more than once? I knew in my soul that cancer was not something that would come back into my body. I made a very conscious decision to do whatever it took to stay healthy.

And let's be honest—I like to keep it simple, so I'm calling this chapter "My Simple and Doable Stay-Healthy Guide." It has two sections: Lifestyle and Diet. After much research and trial and error in my own life, I found that these habits make a huge difference to my well-being. Some changes came easily to me, like adding more vegetables and fruits to my diet. Others are a struggle—it's still hard for me to get all my vitamins in. But I know that I feel better mentally, physically, and emotionally when I make the time to implement my tools, and I hope they will inspire you to create some new rituals in your own life.

MY TOOLBOX

Lifestyle

- Stop and Slow Down
- Get Grounded and Balanced
- Meditation
- Exercise
- Being Happy and Grateful
- Tossing the Toxics

Diet

- Know What to Eat
- Know What to Avoid
- Drink Your Greens
- Up Your Antioxidants
- Get on the Supplement Bandwagon
- My Super-Easy Morning Shake

Just recently I actually stopped in my tracks and said, "Okay, what's going on here? I don't feel like myself." It was one of those days when the to-do list was just too long—it seemed as though nothing was getting crossed off, and everyone needed me to do something for them—the kids needed to be dropped off places, Frank needed me to help at the office, and we were having some work done on the house. It's never just one thing that gets me stressed, but I am learning to deal with stressful situations better. It's times like this that I think about what I can use from my toolbox.

I stopped for a few minutes and reflected. Why was I feeling so out of control and not in balance? Was I exercising? Yes. Was I meditating? No, my schedule was thrown off in summer. Was I practicing gratitude? Yes, but not formally in my book. How was my diet? Was I having a little too much summer fun with ices and barbecues? Probably. Okay, what was I willing to change? I was ready to relax into the new summer schedule, which to me meant being available to my kids and driving them here and there. I would relax and make time to meditate on a more consistent basis. As for the food, I made a conscious commitment to eat more of the very abundant greens from my garden and surrounding farm stands. And I gave myself permission to enjoy all the great things summer has to offer, like an ice here or there, or a scoop of organic ice cream.

The best part about making these lifestyle and dietary changes is the way they make me look. You might wonder; what do they look like? Well, for one my latest blood work showed I am one healthy wellness warrior! I can see changes in my skin, hair, body, and overall glow. The other day as I was leaving the house first thing in the morning to go write, Frank stopped me in the kitchen and said, "Wow, you look so young and happy."

I wasn't dressed up. In fact, my hair was pulled back in a ponytail, and I might have had some lip gloss on. I was just being me. He isn't the only person who has noticed my inner and outer glow. Every time I get a compliment, I smile and say, "Thank you." I like to refer to as myself as "radiating health and wellness." I know you can do it too!

Diet was a crucial area of upgrade for me. The old me ate better than most people. I ate greens, but not on a daily basis. Now I am adamant about getting five servings of greens and fruit every day. I eat whole, real foods, including fruit, greens, and nuts, and I limit the sugar in my life. I challenge people all the time to eat real food and dare them not to feel better. As you read, you will see how I go about doing all that and still live my life in the real world.

I've also started owning my post cancer body and really appreciating all that it has done for me. I've read about and talked to women who had a difficult time dealing with their postsurgical bodies, even years later. I feel so fortunate to be able to own and love my body. All the good healthy food and my overall relaxed attitude have affected my looks for the better! Wow, if that doesn't make me want to continue doing what I doing, I am not sure what will. Who knew that I could or would be better after cancer?

PART 1: LIFESTYLE

The biggest question people ask me is how I've changed since cancer. I can't answer that in simple words. Many things have changed. One of the biggest changes is my attitude toward my body. The experience of having a portion of my body operated on has taught me to appreciate every part of it—the parts I love and the parts I don't. I am also much more present in my life. I say yes more often to the things I want to do and no to the things I don't want to do. I really appreciate and seek out time to be with my kids and husband. I love having an active role in their lives. I enjoy reading with them, talking with them, spending time with them, cooking with them, and more. I constantly remind myself not to sweat the small stuff. So what if the laundry is still in laundry baskets? Or the house needs to be cleaned or I didn't return e-mails? Life still goes on. I want life to go on with me, and for that to happen, it means I need to let things go.

I've also decided to surround myself with people who think and act more like me. I want to be around happy, positive people. I took the time to look deep within myself to learn how to change negative thoughts and become a calmer, more balanced person. I figured ways to add meditation, yoga, and more grounding activities into my daily life.

TIP 1: STOP AND SLOW DOWN

One of the biggest changes I've made is slowing down my life. Making a green juice or smoothie or staying away from processed food is easy for me. I would rank asking me to slow down at a difficulty level of 10. I used to "run" at 120 mph each day. I would run from one activity to another. I started by letting go of my huge, ongoing to-do list and crossing things off it. Now I make time in my calendar to include downtime even if it's only thirty minutes of quiet time.

I take things at a much slower pace these days by using different tricks to help myself slow down. One is running. Okay, I know that sounds like an oxymoron, but it's really not. Running helps me stay in the present moment. Yoga is another activity that helps me stay present and keep my mind in check. Yoga reinforces the practice of the here and now.

I learned to hit the stop button and reevaluate what is working at this moment and what is not working. Sometimes just making time for an extra yoga class helps rebalance, and sometimes it means an overnight visit to a hotel alone to "escape." I would have never thought of leaving Frank and the kids to escape overnight for a chance to be alone; and I even feel guilty admitting to it. But I have seen the benefits of stopping and regrouping. I know how my body and mind feel when I am in balance, and I know when I'm off. The trick is practicing this on a daily basis to ensure I'm not out of balance for too long.

I've stopped comparing myself with everyone else. I volunteer with several community groups, and instead of going full force with activities or chairing the new project, I hang back now. I realize that I work better at a much slower, more deliberate pace, not a pace that will stress me out. I have also learned how to stay away from things that upset me. If I am not having fun and enjoying the people I am working with, I just don't do it. Frank reminds me that when I volunteer for these activities, I am not being paid and that nobody has the ability to fire me!

TAKEAWAY: SLOW DOWN

1. Find tricks to help you slow down each day.
2. Stop rushing from place to place and make time in your daily calendar for downtime.
3. Use yoga or running or whatever works for you to help stay in the present moment.
4. Learn how to say no and feel good about it.

TIP 2: GET GROUNDED AND BALANCED

Staying grounded to me means enjoying the moment and having gratitude for what is going on around me. Unfortunately, this can be a struggle. I am constantly working on it. I told you some of the rituals were easier for me than others!

I have learned how to sit with my thoughts and be in tune with my mind and body. I wait and listen for the answers. In my experience, the answers don't come in a voice from above but are more like guidance about what I should do next. I learned that stopping and doing nothing is an opportunity for me to reconnect with some power higher than me. That higher power can be God, an angel, or guides; for me it's all three.

I try to stay in the moment, because even a simple drop-off at a karate or dance class can get old fast. When I'm not in the moment, I get anxious about getting stuck at the railroad crossing or behind a school bus. I am lucky I have my three kids to help me stay on task with relaxing. All three of them call me out when they see me getting annoyed at things around me.

Being able to keep yourself functioning optimally means knowing what's working and being able to say what isn't working. As I write, I remember that when Frank and I taught marriage preparation classes, we used a workbook called *A Decision to Love.* We would remind our students that it had that name for a reason. Love doesn't always come easily, and sometimes on a very conscious level you need to make the decision to love your partner. It's the same for loving yourself and keeping yourself in balance. Sometimes the decision to love myself means cancelling a class I was supposed to teach because I just don't have the energy, or maybe it's saying no to friends who are going out for drinks or simply hitting delete on an email because I know it's just going to annoy me.

Takeaway: Being in Balance

1. Find out what being in balance means to you.
2. Enjoy being in the now and take time to do nothing
3. Get others to help you relax and not sweat the small stuff.
4. Decide to love yourself and choose the actions that support you best.

Tip 3: Meditation

For me, meditation is about taking the time to just stop, breathe, and regroup. I think of it as an opportunity to clean my mind, kind of like hitting the TiVo delete button with the little "bleep-bleep" sound and all. Sometimes my meditation can be a whole sixty seconds and other times it can be twenty-five minutes. I strive for about fifteen minutes a day.

This practice has helped me learn how to let go physically of things that bother me. It helps my body and mind calm down at the same time. I am constantly reminded how much my body holds on to thoughts. If something is bothering me, such as an upcoming doctor visit, I have learned to acknowledge the fear. But I let the fear move through my body instead of manifesting itself in my body. The idea behind my meditation is that my fears are present, acknowledged, released, and then replaced with a positive message of strength.

The "how" of meditation is not important: you can do it on a cushion, lying in bed, or just sitting in the car. I meditate in the car while waiting for the kids to come out of a class or while I'm sitting quietly in my backyard. I try to meditate when it's time to regroup my thoughts so I'm not just rushing from one kid to pick up to another. I find it very useful when I feel myself getting frustrated in the long supermarket line or when I need it most—sitting in traffic! My kids also help me gauge when I'm feeling agitated. I am so lucky to have them be the voice of reason. They help me stop my mind from racing and remind me that being late is okay sometimes. Boy, how lucky am I?

MY SIX-STEP MEDITATION METHOD:

1. Breathe deeply from your abdomen. Put one hand on your chest and the other on your abdomen. Now focus on the hand on the abdomen and let that hand rise and fall with your deep breaths.
2. Start letting your breath travel down your whole body.
3. Now imagine white light entering your body from the top of your head. Let that light travel through your body and really tune in to the healing power of the light traveling down.
4. Release in your mind any thoughts that aren't serving you to be your best self. Imagine those thoughts being released through the root of your spine.
5. Acknowledge any thoughts that are coming up, welcome them, and set them free. It's amazing what thoughts come up when you're meditating. The idea is to let the thoughts come up, feel them, and then set them free.
6. The last step is to replace the thoughts that don't serve you with more positive healing thoughts.

Takeaway: Meditation

1. Take time to breathe deeply with deep abdominal breathing.
2. Allow your body to acknowledge things that are bothering you.
3. Mentally release thoughts that aren't serving your best interest.
4. Incorporate good healing thoughts on a daily basis even if it's just for a few moments.

Tip 4: Exercise

One of the main reasons I exercise is obviously to stay healthy and fit. Study after study shows the positive effects of exercise, specifically for cancer survivors. Exercise, like meditation, helps boost the immune system. It also assists with hormone balance and has the ability to reduce excess estrogen and testosterone that stimulates the growth of cancers, especially breast cancer, according to research from the *Journal of Nutrition*. One doctor in Paris even prescribes exercise as part of chemotherapy treatments. Dr. Bouillet says that when his patients were physically active, they had distinctly fewer relapses than other cancer patients, according to the *Anticancer* book.

You've probably heard of runner's high. Well, when you exercise, your body releases chemicals called endorphins, which trigger a positive feeling in the body and help with anxiety, depression, and stress. I am continually amazed that my body can do what it does. When I'm out on a long run, I can work things out in my head that I haven't been able to get answers to otherwise. Hey, I'm not saying I solve all my problems with running, but great thoughts usually occur. I love repeating my mantra while running: "Running makes me feel strong and healthy." Running forces me to stay in the moment and not think about how many more miles I have left. Whether I go out for three miles or ten, I force myself to just keep running and stop my mind from saying, "Oh no, I have nine more miles left!" Keeping that mind-set definitely takes practice.

Another reason I love running is that it gets me out in nature. I don't run on a treadmill. I run outside year-round. I love feeling the fresh air on my face and tuning in to the trees swaying around me. I even started trail running, so I actually run through the woods and forgo the sidewalk.

In 2013 I wanted to take my running up a notch, so I signed up to do the ultimate run: a marathon. My goal was to cross the finish line with a big smile across my face and I did. I was uncomfortable at times, but I knew deep down I could do it. After beating cancer I feel like I can do anything I set my mind to.

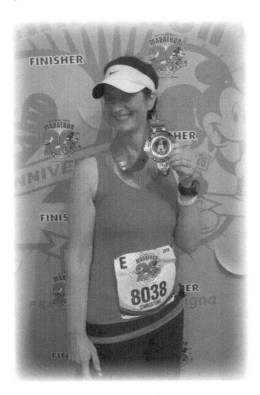

Me right after finishing the Disney marathon.

Three important factors have helped me maintain an exercise routine: exercising with friends, having fun and setting goals. I've found that exercising with a buddy or a group keeps me motivated. Whether I'm meeting a friend at yoga class or just going out for a run with Frank, I know I have to show up. I can't just skip it. When I trained for my marathon, I trained with a running group. Could I have run on my own? Yes, but running with a group made the process more fun. We didn't all run at the same rate—some were faster, some were slower—but the idea is that we met as a group to do something healthy together. Similar to enjoying the good, healthy foods every day, maintaining a regular exercise schedule has to be enjoyable. Spending time in nature, listening to inspirational music, and feeling great afterward keep it fun for me. Finally, in order to stay with a routine, I have to attach goals to the program. So when I participated in kickboxing, I entered a contest to see who could improve their fitness level and body mass index. It was great to track my progress and compete with other people in the class. Although I didn't win the final contest, I kept with it for the 12 weeks of the contest and even a little afterward.

TAKEAWAY: EXERCISE

1. Exercise is great for your body: it strengthens your heart muscle, lowers blood pressure, and reduces body fat.
2. Exercise helps your body release endorphins, which can help fight depression, stress, and anxiety.
3. Find an exercise you love and start small. Try a ten-minute walk and work your way to thirty minutes, and start reaping the benefits.
4. Get a friend to walk with you.

TIP 5: BEING HAPPY AND GRATEFUL

I recently watched a TED Talk about happiness. In the twelve-minute video, author and lecturer Shawn Anchor highlights what it takes to be happy. While I was watching this video, I realized that during my year of cancer treatment, I was unconsciously doing many of the things on his list!

He says the first way to create lasting positive change is to write down three things for which you are grateful each day. My practice of recalling at least three positive events that happened in a day helped redirect my mind to recall the good things instead of the annoying ones. Some of my gratitudes were as simple as no traffic on the way to treatment, making a great-tasting smoothie that I enjoyed, or just hanging out with the kids. The gratitude list helped me re-create the simple pleasures in the day.

Science backs me up here. Robert Emmons, PhD, and Mike McCollough studied gratitude and reported their research in the *Journal of Personality and Social Psychology*. They found people who wrote down five things that they were grateful for in a week felt better about their lives as a whole and were 25 percent happier than those who listed five events that hassled them. The happier group also reported fewer health complaints. I figured that recalling things for which I am grateful was a great way to improve my health.

I found a way of transforming my daily gratitude from thoughts into words. I met Lorraine Miller, author of *From Gratitude to Bliss: A Journey in Health and Happiness*, at a nutrition conference. Her book is a step-by-step guide to incorporating gratitude into your daily life. In it, she includes inspiring tips on keeping a positive mind-set. The book was a great starting point for me to really practice gratitude. Although I was listing my gratitudes in my head at night before bed, I got into the habit of writing them down in my new gratitude journal from Lorraine. Keeping this journal also helped me focus on the goodness in my life during a time when it was easy to find darkness and unhappiness. The idea of writing down my daily gratitudes helped me look at the bigger picture in life, not just my current situation.

One of the gratitudes I wrote down was when I was going through radiation and running a six-mile race. Yes, you read that correctly. My race pace had dropped to a slow crawl, but instead of being upset that I was barely even running, I took the opportunity to talk with the people around me. I was running next to a man at mile five who had run a race every weekend for the last sixteen years! I was disappointed that I was running so slowly, but here was this veteran runner who was running at my pace. Meeting him helped me reframe my thoughts from disappointment to being happy that I finished the race. If I had been running my regular pace, I never would have talked with him. Pretty cool, right?

Shawn Anchor also says that journaling is a way to create lasting happiness. Journaling about even one positive thing that happened within the past twenty-four hours allows your brain to relive the happiness. Although I did not keep a daily journal during my treatment, I did blog about my positive experiences.

Anchor says that meditation allows your mind to focus on the task at hand and is another way of retraining your mind toward happiness. I used meditation during my yoga classes and in my therapy sessions. My ten to fifteen minutes of meditation helps me stay in the present, clears my head of any scary, negative thoughts, and helps bring good healing thoughts to my body.

Another person I turned to who teaches about happiness and gratitude is Tony Robbins, self-help author and motivational speaker. He says, "When you are grateful, fear disappears." He explains that a person cannot be in gratitude and in a fearful state of mind at the same time. I felt as though Tony's quote spoke to me, so I posted it on my mirror in my bathroom and on my phone. I even repeated it in my head while I was undergoing treatments. His quote makes me stop and remember what I am grateful for in each moment.

Tony Robbins also loves to ask, "What story are you telling yourself?" Are you telling yourself over and over again that you are a victim of cancer? Are you telling yourself that cancer will come back? Are you stuck in the role of being sick? These questions and stories can come up for all us. I have made a very conscious decision to tell myself I am a healthy person and that my "story" is not one of cancer but of health and wellness. What story do you want to tell?

The last tool for training your brain to become more positive, according to Anchor, is to practice random acts of kindness. When you share your positive behavior, it creates a ripple effect to those around you. When I listened to this part of the video, I had a huge smile on my face. I was thinking about the sticky notes I left in the dressing room at my radiation treatments. I was passing my positive thoughts on to others around me. Finding the best quotes and leaving them on the mirror gave me something to look forward to every day during radiation. Not only was I inspiring myself, but I hoped it brought a smile to someone else.

TAKEAWAY:

1. Write down three things you are grateful for each day.
2. Journal about one positive thing each day.
3. Decide what "story" you want to tell yourself.
4. Remember that when you feel gratitude, fear disappears.
5. Practice random acts of kindness.

Tip 7: Tossing the Toxics

Once I started really cleaning up my diet, I started thinking about all the chemicals I came in contact with every day and specifically, the chemicals that had been linked to cancer. I evaluated my morning routine, starting with my shower: the body soap, shampoo, and conditioner. After my shower, I would layer on skin lotion, face lotion, and hair products. Next came the antiperspirant and the makeup. Were all my products safe to use? I turned to the Internet to do some major research. Two websites helped me gather information: the Environmental Working Group (www.ewg.org) and the Glamorganic Goddess (www.theglamorganicgoddess.blogspot.com). Both sites helped me determine which products would lessen the amount of toxins I took in. Danielle Messina, who is known as the Glamorganic Goddess, also has a connection to breast cancer. She started her blog to help herself and others sort out which natural and organic products had the least toxic chemicals and performed well enough to use. Looking at ingredients lists and researching products can be exhausting and overwhelming, especially when a chemical can be listed on a product twenty different ways.

But I found some obvious chemicals that needed to get out of my life and would like to share them with you.

1. **Plastic**

The first toxic material I addressed was plastic. The potential problem with plastic is that it contains a chemical called Bispenol-a or BPA, which has been shown to leach into the bloodstream, affecting hormone levels. Researchers from Indiana University studied how BPA may be more easily absorbed by breast tumor cells than healthy cells. "BPA very likely plays a role in disrupting the normal metabolic balance of hormone-sensitive tissues and organs," according to health advocate Mike Adams in a NaturalNews. com article. I realized how many things in my house contained BPA—and it wasn't just plastic items, but some canned items too. I replaced plastic drinking bottles with stainless steel or glass. I like to think of myself as plastic-free. I walk around with my glass drinking bottle, and I use a glass straw to drink my smoothies. The few plastic food containers I have are for nonfood items now. When I have leftover food, it goes into a glass storage container. I still eat beans from a can, but the brand I use is BPA-free.

2. **Parabens**

Another chemical I wanted out of my house was parabens. They sound innocent enough as a preservative found in common personal care items such as shampoo, lotions, soap, sunscreens, and makeup. The problem with parabens, like BPA, is that they mimic estrogen in the body and have been found in breast cancer tumors. As I was writing this book, a new study done in the United Kingdom showed that nearly every woman with breast cancer has one or more paraben chemicals in her breast tissue, suggesting a possible link between the chemical and the disease. Dr. Philippa Darbre and her team found that 99 percent of breast cancer tissue samples contained at least one type of paraben, and 60 percent contained at least five. Although my tissue sample was not tested for parabens, I wanted to avoid them at all costs. I started researching all of my health and beauty aid products, only to realize the skin lotion I had used for years to keep my skin soft and hydrated clearly listed parabens as one of its ingredients. I was devastated that this lotion had the ability to penetrate my skin, enter my bloodstream, and disrupt my estrogen levels. It made my stomach sick to think that the lotion I was putting on my skin every day to keep it moisturized contained parabens.

It didn't happen overnight, but I am now vigilant about the products I use. It takes time to read labels and be sure if the product is free of the chemical *and* if I actually like how it works. The Glamorganic Goddess site was helpful, and the perfect place for me to start. I now make my own body and face lotion. I never thought I would become one of those people who make their own products, but I love how my skin feels. I mix coconut oil (from the kitchen) with some drops of Young Living Oils. Coconut oil is antimicrobial, antifungal, antibacterial, and antioxidant, and leaves my skin feeling so smooth. I also changed my daily soap to Dr. Bronner's brand.

3. **Phthalates**

Parabens aren't the only toxic chemicals found in my personal care items. I also started to learn about phthalates—another group of endocrine-disrupting chemicals. According to the EWG's website, phthalates are a group of industrial chemicals used to make plastics more flexible as well as solvents. I soon realized I was surrounded by them: in toys, food packaging, hoses, shower curtains, vinyl floor coverings, lubricants, adhesives, detergents, nail polish, shampoo, and hairspray. I looked for labels that said "phthalate-free" and made sure my laundry detergent didn't include this chemical along with my shampoo or conditioner. I make sure the personal care products I buy don't list DBP and DEP or BzBP. I avoid products that list "fragrance" as an ingredient, because that fragrance could include one of the chemicals listed above.

4. **Perflurooctaniod Acid**

The next chemical I needed out of my life was Perflurooctaniod Acid (PFOA). According to the EWG, PFOA can be found in nonstick pans, furniture, cosmetics, household cleaners, and clothing as well as packaged-food containers. Okay, so this is extremely difficult to completely avoid, because it is just part of our environment. But I did what I could by replacing my nonstick cookware with stainless steel cookware. I switched my household cleaners to brands that don't use toxic chemicals, or made my own using vinegar and water. I avoid anything that says "stain-resistant." I look for the ingredient "fluoro" or "perfluoro" in products such as nail polish, moisturizers, makeup, and other personal care items.

Once I realized I was exposed to more than one hundred chemicals every day, I made a conscious effect to limit the ones I had an opportunity to change. Ultimately, it's really up to you to decide if you are happy with the results from each product you use.

Takeaway: Top Eight Things I Do to Detoxify My Life

1. I make sure people remove their shoes when they enter my house, limiting the amount of toxic environmental toxins dragged in.
2. I changed my shampoo/conditioner/laundry detergent to be sure they were made with natural ingredients that I trusted.
3. I put in a water purifying system so I didn't need to purchase plastic water bottles, and I drink only from glass bottles.
4. I pulled up my stain-resistant carpets and replaced them with natural-fiber area rugs.
5. I avoided the use of chemical fertilizers on the lawn or in the garden

6. I got rid of my nonstick pans (Teflon) and slowly replaced them with stainless steel.
7. I switched my skin and face moisturizer to coconut oil.
8. I replaced my makeup with a nonchemical, 100 percent fruit-pigmented brand.

PART 2: DIET

I feel lucky when it comes to the food portion of an anticancer lifestyle. I was already eating pretty healthy even before the big C. The main point I want to make when it comes to food is really simple: *eat real food!* I love food writer Michael Pollan's quote, "Don't eat anything that your great-grandmother would not recognize as food."

Think about that for a moment. Would your great-grandmother recognize brightly colored yogurt from a squeeze package, or chicken that has been processed and pressed into different shapes? I doubt it. She would recognize fruits, veggies, and whole chickens.

When I first started transitioning to whole foods, I looked at labels and realized how much food I ate from packages that listed more than five ingredients. I was amazed to see the cereal I was eating had a ton of added ingredients, so I switched to steel-cut oats: just one ingredient. I added my own fruits to my oatmeal and realized how much better I felt.

Transitioning to healthier foods reminds me of when I started training for my marathon. In the beginning, 26.1 miles was far beyond what I thought I was capable of running. So I broke it down to make it seem achievable. Step one was planning my runs. I actually set up a calendar with my daily runs and the mileage. Every week I slowly built up my mileage. I didn't just go out and run the twenty-six miles. I took it slowly, added mileage each week, and took my time and enjoyed the runs. I set myself up with a coach and surrounded myself with people who could help me achieve this milestone.

The same can be said about food. I didn't just throw away and ban all cookies, pastas, and pretzels from my house (that's not the best thing to do when you have three kids). I started slowly making small changes. I added salads to meals, and filled the house with a variety of fruits, nuts, and seeds for snacking. I replaced everyday food with healthier foods. I made my own salad dressing, and then added a variety of raw vegetables to my salad. I made homemade soups and added chopped-up greens to make them even healthier. I started making smoothies and juices. I started slowly with juices too. I added more fruit than greens and worked my way up to mostly green juices. I used the same process for the other changes I made in my life: stress reduction, meditation, gratitude, and removal of toxins.

It sounds simple, right? I think about eating real whole foods: whole pieces of fruit (not from a can or plastic container), fresh veggies (not in a can) and small quantities of high-quality meat (organic).

TIP 1: KNOW WHAT TO EAT

In my journey I turned to many different books, doctors, and research papers that explain how food can be just as powerful as medication. That idea of food as medicine really appealed to me. I had control over what I was putting into my body, and eating was something I did every day, several times a day.

The main food I increased was green vegetables. I'm not going to go into all the research behind the benefits of eating greens, because you already know you need to eat more veggies. The green vegetables in particular are packed with vitamins and minerals needed to keep your body strong both during treatments and post treatment. Green vegetables should become your new go-to food. Think of green veggies as the energy of life; when you add them to your life, you have energy!

I was taught about the power of greens at the Institute for Integrative Nutrition. I can't pick up a newspaper or magazine that doesn't have an article talking about green vegetables being the most powerful food, never mind the best anti–breast cancer food. According to Dr. Joel Fuhrman's website, "Close to 300 case-controlled studies show a protective effect of vegetable consumption against cancer and that cruciferous vegetables are the foods with the most powerful anti-cancer effects of all foods. While eating fresh fruits, beans, vegetables, seeds and nuts have been all been shown in scientific studies to reduce occurrence of cancer, cruciferous vegetables are different. Instead of a 1 to 1 relationship they have 1 to 2 relationship with a wide variety of human cancers."

When I saw Dr. Fuhrman speak at a nutrition conference in 2011 he explained it quite simply by saying, "When plant food intake goes up by 20 percent in a group, cancer rates typically drop by 20 percent and with cruciferous vegetables cancer rates drop by 40 percent."

Other research shows the protective effects of broccoli sprouts against breast cancer. In a 2012 GreenMedInfo.com article, Dr. Veronique Desaulniers explains their distinct value, specifically talking about the compound sulforaphane and how it's been found to cause cancer cell death and decrease the expression of estrogen receptors.

The one green that I add to as many meals as possible is kale. It's the powerhouse of greens. Kale is part of the cruciferous family (a.k.a. the cabbage family), which has special cancer-fighting properties, and it includes vitamins A, C, and K and omega-3 fatty acids. This super dark leafy veggie can be found at the local supermarket, not just farmers' markets or farm stands.

If eating kale is too much of a leap for you to take, then start with spinach. Spinach is a tasty green that can easily be put into foods without your even knowing it's there. When I first started eating more healthfully, I started adding small amounts of spinach leaves to salads. I would sneak some spinach leaves onto a sandwich along with other lettuce. I would cut spinach up into small pieces and add it to a pasta dish. The way I started eating spinach is the same way I started incorporating kale into my daily diet. I found it important not to go all in at one time. I made the transition slowly. By adding the healthful greens into my daily diet slowly, I let my taste buds adjust to their different tastes and textures.

I am a big believer in eating the highest-quality fruits and vegetables available. That means taking advantage of what my local farmer has to offer. By eating local farm-fresh organic food, I am eating food that is in season and available immediately without being shipped across the country. The foods produced locally are more nutrient dense because they are eaten right after they are picked from the farm. I belong to a Community Supported Agriculture program (CSA) called the Golden Earthworm. They are a certified organic farm that produces food for the community to enjoy. The farm feeds us year-round. My family and I literally know the farmers who feed us on a daily basis. I make meals and create menu plans with whatever food is harvested that week at the farm.

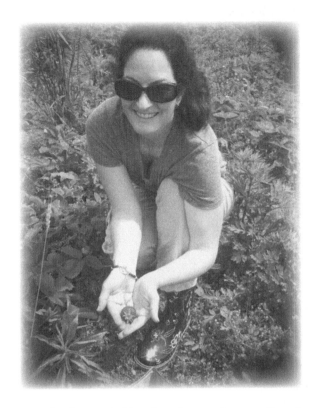

Me at the farm picking local organic strawberries.

I decided that if I was eating all these extra vegetables and fruits every day, I wanted to be sure they were of the highest quality. For me that meant eating mostly organic fruits and vegetables. Sometimes organic can cost a little more, but to me it is money well spent. I put enough poison into my body with the low-dose chemotherapy and radiation; I don't want to add to it with pesticides and other residue from nonorganic foods. When I was in nutrition school, I learned about two important lists. One, called the Dirty Dozen, lists the produce most likely to contain the most harmful chemicals because of pesticides. The other list is called the "Clean 15." These lists highlights foods with the lowest pesticide load, and are the safest conventionally grown crops to consume from the standpoint of pesticide contamination. These lists are updated each year, so you can always go to www.ewg.org for the latest info.

2012 Dirty Dozen

1. Apples
2. Celery
3. Sweet bell peppers
4. Peaches
5. Strawberries
6. Nectarines (imported)
7. Grapes
8. Spinach
9. Lettuce
10. Cucumbers
11. Blueberries (domestic)
12. Potatoes

2012 Clean 15

1. Onions
2. Sweet corn
3. Pineapples
4. Avocado
5. Cabbage
6. Sweet peas
7. Asparagus
8. Mangoes
9. Eggplant
10. Kiwi
11. Cantaloupe (domestic)
12. Sweet potatoes
13. Grapefruit
14. Watermelon
15. Mushrooms

I love the simple idea that I have control over what is going into my body. I consciously choose foods that support my immune system and prevent tumors from creating inflammation that can feed cancer cells. I seek out foods that promote the suicide of cancer cells. And the beauty of it all is that these foods taste amazing.

TAKEAWAY: EAT YOUR WHOLE FOODS

1. Start eating whole foods or foods that your grandmother would recognize.
2. Cruciferous vegetables are the most powerful anticancer foods; think broccoli, kale, cabbage, bok choy, and other green leafy vegetables.
3. Start adding spinach to your meals, working your way up to the powerhouse green vegetable: kale.
4. Switch to organic fruits and vegetables. Use the Dirty Dozen and the Clean 15 lists to help guide you.
5. Investigate eating local farm-fresh food by joining a Community Supported Agriculture program. Check out www.localharvest. org/csa.

TIP 2: KNOW WHAT TO AVOID

Are there really foods that can promote cancer growth? In doing research for my own diet, I turned to Dr. David Servan-Schreiber, author of *Anticancer: A New Way of Life,* and Suzanne Boothby, author of *The After Cancer Diet.* Both authors look at how different foods can actually promote the growth of cancer cells.

Servan-Schreiber says in his book that there are actual anticancer foods. "If certain foods in our diet can act as fertilizers for tumors, others, to the contrary, harbor precious anticancer molecules," he writes.

He goes on to say that all the scientific literature points in the same direction: people who want to protect themselves from cancer should seriously reduce their consumption of processed sugar and bleached flour.

So what did this mean to me? It relates to Michael Pollan's quote about eating real food. When I eat real food in its natural form, I avoid eating processed sugar and bleached flour.

I was looking for more information about sugar and why it needs to be avoided. Boothby explains in her book that for every bit of sugar you eat, you are losing nutrients and promoting inflammation. She explains the hard truth about sugar: every time you eat even a small piece of candy, you could be helping to grow a new tumor or promote abnormal cell growth. "Foods high on the glycemic index cause the body to secrete insulin and insulin-like growth factor (IGF)," she writes. "These hormones promote cell growth and inflammation, inhibiting the body's natural defenses against developing cancer."

I like how she explains inflammation as a silent ongoing, chronic condition that you can't feel. "If you don't have a great diet, you don't have room to consume excess sugar," she says. Boothby explains that sugar is hidden in many foods today, so she suggests that people transition slowly, staying away from processed foods and adding more whole foods.

I know the idea of avoiding sugar entirely might seem a little out there, but here's what I've done to reduce my intake. Before cancer, I might have absentmindedly snacked on cookies throughout the day. Now I have stronger intentions. I've upgraded my snacks to nuts and seeds, and I always have fresh apples and almond butter on hand.

If I do have dessert, I make sure it's the highest quality possible and tastes really good. I don't waste my sweet tooth on a bite of something from a box or a bag. I go to a top-quality bakery and pick out something truly delicious.

I also make my own desserts with ingredients I enjoy. I've started making homemade ice cream with raw milk and a touch of honey, and let me tell you, it's divine. You might be thinking that making your own ice cream is over the top—that's what I thought—but after doing it once, I realized it doesn't take much time and is totally worth it.

TAKEAWAY: WHAT TO AVOID

1. Get the sugar out of your diet!
2. Stay away from processed food—anything from a box that may have hidden sugar.
3. Be intentional with your snacking, and truly enjoy the desserts you choose to eat.

TIP 3: DRINK YOUR GREENS

Plain and simple, more greens = better health. Okay, so what did that mean to me? I thought I was getting enough green veggies with a salad and whatever vegetable was in season. But now that I am on the super-healthy track, I am committed to eating as many green veggies as possible each day. I figured out that for me, the simplest way to include all the benefits that greens have to offer is to have them at every meal. I started making smoothies and green juices.

I had always read about adding more greens to my diet, and I did it here and there, but now I have greens *every day*. Wow, what a difference it made in my life! I did a little food experiment. I included a green smoothie or juice every day for fourteen days straight. Guess what? I felt great. My energy levels were high, and I didn't crash at four o'clock. And if I forgot to drink my greens for the day, I was dragging in the afternoon, a little crabby, and probably looking for something that was not in my best interest (usually something sweet). Including more green vegetables on a daily basis not only helped my body get a ton of vitamins and minerals, and increase my energy levels, but reduced my sugar cravings.

I love how great I feel after drinking a smoothie or juice. I feel energetic, my mind is clear, and I'm less crabby. My skin looks clear and my hair is shiny, so the drinks literally affect me inside and out. If I didn't love how great the smoothies or shakes made me feel, I would find it difficult to stick with them on a daily basis.

The first green smoothie I made had a handful of spinach and a cut-up apple blended with some water. I saw this green, thick-looking sludge. Yuck! I couldn't drink it. It just tasted too "green" for me. I realized I needed to slowly jump into the world of blending my vegetables. I didn't give up. Instead I researched the best fruit-to-greens ratio for beginners. I realized that I had to give my taste buds an opportunity to adjust to the taste of blending raw greens. I learned to add three fruits to every handful of raw greens. The next green shake I made included a fistful of spinach, two apples, and lots of pineapple. I loved it. I soon realized that these smoothies were a simple way for me to get extra greens (and fruit) into my diet, in addition to meals. Now I can make great-tasting smoothies in my sleep. It has become my passion to introduce people to drinking their greens.

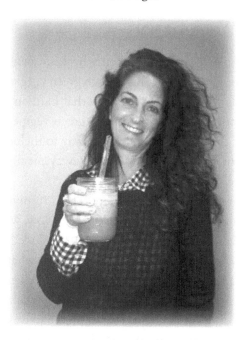

My daily smoothie in my glass jar with my glass straw.

Once I got my smoothies down, I decided to check out juicing. When I first purchased a juicer, it sat on my counter for more than a week before I actually used it. I had no idea how many vegetables to use, which fruits were best, or how to clean the machine when I was finished. I finally got the courage to experiment. After all, it was just a juicer! Again, I started slowly; using vegetables that I knew contained high water content: cucumber and celery. Then I started adding in raw greens: spinach and kale. I finished off the juice with various fruits: grapefruit, pineapple, apples, or pears. Before I knew it, not only was I enjoying juicing, but my family was enjoying it too. My youngest, Jack, is my juicing assistant. He loves pushing the foods down the juicing chute. Now, if I could just get one of the kids to help me clean up!

WHAT'S THE DIFFERENCE BETWEEN A SMOOTHIE AND JUICE?

The big difference between my smoothies and my juice is the amount of vegetables I use. When I juice, I use more vegetables and fruit. The type of juicer I have is called a "masticator." My husband (the orthodontist) got the biggest kick out of me purchasing a juicer that actually "chews" the

100

food that is put through the juicer chute. The juicer takes the fiber out of the fruits and vegetables. When I use the juicer, I'm left with a nutritionally potent, thin liquid.

When I make a smoothie, the texture is a little thicker because the plant fiber is present, which also makes them more filling. Something else I learned is that since the whole plant is blended, not juiced, my body works a bit harder to digest a smoothie and absorb the nutrients. Some juicing experts say that your body absorbs the nutrients from a juice within ten minutes of drinking, calling it the ultimate fast food.

My favorite tip to share with newbies is to include lemon, lime, or ginger. Or, if you are super adventurous, try all three! These ingredients will seriously add a *wow* factor to any smoothie or juice.

TAKEAWAY:

1. Experiment with blending green vegetables and fruit into a smoothie.
2. Do an experiment and see how your body feels after drinking the smoothie.
3. Order a "green juice" at your local health food store, and have them add more fruit if it's your first-ever green drink.
4. Add lemon, ginger, and/or lime to enhance the flavor of your smoothie or juice.

TIP 4: UP YOUR ANTIOXIDANTS

I'd heard the word *antioxidants* before, but in order to explain what they are in simple terms, I turned to Dr. Edward Group, founder of the Global Healing Center, one of the one of the largest alternative, natural, and organic health resources on the Internet. He compares antioxidants to the bottom-feeder fish in a fish tank; they are eating all the gunk and grime that is toxic for the rest of the fish. Antioxidants are the molecular-sized "free radical scavengers" in the fish tank of your body. Simple, right? Antioxidants = good things.

I was taught in nutrition school that eating antioxidants helps slow down the oxidation of free radicals. Dr. Group says that free radicals create a destructive process in our cells, causing the molecules within the cells to become unstable. Free radicals are unstable, and in order to become more stable, they attack other healthy cells. He goes on to say that free radicals are bullies that start pushing everybody around and encourage nice cells to become bullies as well. The results are "free radical waste products" made up of our broken, injured, and deformed cells. If our cells are weak, it is natural that our organs, tissues, and skin will likewise become weakened.

I found it simply amazing that all this was going on within my body. I wanted to be sure that antioxidants were part of my daily diet, but what did that mean. I soon realized it meant that I stayed on the same path I was already on—eating whole foods in a range colors. Dr. Mark Hyman is family physician and a bestselling health and wellness author. Here's his list of the top antioxidant-rich foods.

Top 20 Antioxidant Foods

1. Small red beans, dried
2. Wild blueberries
3. Red kidney beans
4. Pinto beans
5. Blueberries, cultivated
6. Cranberries
7. Artichokes, cooked
8. Blackberries
9. Prunes
10. Raspberries
11. Strawberries
12. Red Delicious apples
13. Granny Smith apples
14. Pecans
15. Sweet cherries
16. Black plums
17. Russet potatoes, cooked
18. Black beans
19. Plums

It is really pretty amazing that the top antioxidant fruits not only taste great, but are seasonal as well. Strawberries start in late spring, followed by raspberries, blueberries, and blackberries. By summertime cherries and plums are in season too. In the fall apples and pears are ready to be picked. I just love when nature provides. It was obvious to me yet again that the food aspect of health is quite simple. Eat whole foods and eat them in season.

In *Anticancer*, Servan-Schreiber writes about the power of raspberries:

> Richard Beliveau, PhD, a researcher in biochemistry and professor at the University of Montreal, runs one of the largest laboratories for molecular medicine in the world specializing in cancer biology. Dr. Beliveau has shown that raspberries have been shown to be just as effective as medication proven to slow the growth of blood vessels. He says if this discovery had been a pharmaceutical molecule, his fax machine would have been going all day and the grants would have been pouring in. But because you can't put a patent on a raspberry, no grants are to be had, and pharmaceutical companies aren't interested.

I included antioxidant-rich foods in my daily diet during all my treatments. But during radiation, I stopped taking all my vitamins and supplements. Let me explain why. Radiation therapy is based on cellular damage; your body is creating free radicals, but in a purposeful way. The goal of radiation treatment is to make free radicals, and the goal of antioxidants is to neutralize free radicals. It made sense to me that if I was committing to the radiation, I would do everything to be sure it worked optimally.

TIPS FOR SUCCESS: ADDING ANTIOXIDANTS

1. Add antioxidant-rich foods to your diet.
2. Create a contest with yourself to see how many you can eat in a day.
3. Tune in to how your body feels after eating whole foods.
4. Be sure to talk to your radiologist about your vitamin and supplements before you start radiation.

TIP 5: GET ON THE SUPPLEMENT BANDWAGON

Another big part of my diet includes taking vitamins and supplements on a daily basis. The recommendations came from two of my doctors. I like to use two separate doctors and bounce ideas off both of them. Both doctors use a variety of tests before making any changes in the supplements I take. The tests may involve how I feel along with blood test results and urine and saliva tests.

I take these vitamins and minerals on a daily basis to help my immunity, keep my body in balance, and keep my "high" estrogen levels in check. Some are easier to literally swallow than others! I have devised ways of ensuring I get them daily. I put all my supplements into a little dish in the morning so, they are altogether and easier to keep track of. Some days I take all of them at once, but most days, I hate swallowing them at one sitting, so I break it up throughout the day. I try to group the smaller pills together (like vitamin D and curcumin) and swallow them as a group, but some others are too large and I need to take them separately. As you can figure, taking a fist full of supplements is something I struggle with, but I understand that they are just one of the puzzle pieces in my goal of staying healthy.

BROCCOLI PILL

Okay, so this one goes against my belief that if I eat well enough, my body should be fine. When my doctor prescribed what I call my broccoli pill, I hesitated and said, "Wait a minute; I can increase my broccoli eating." She explained that I would need to eat more than one hundred pounds of broccoli to get the equivalent of one broccoli pill. All right! I get it. I can eat broccoli, but as a breast cancer thriver, it is important for me to include a daily broccoli pill. Remember, studies show that cruciferous veggies (such as broccoli) are the most powerful anticancer foods. So I smile while I swallow my two broccoli pills daily, knowing all that goodness is going into my body!

VITAMIN D3

Another supplement I'm on is D3. Studies show again and again the importance of vitamin D for our health. Many researchers now believe that vitamin D3 contributes to slowing down all forms of cancer, at least in the early stages.

But I really love what Dr. Joel Fuhrman says about recent research on vitamin D in his book *Super Immunity*: "If Vitamin D supplements were a drug, and if a drug was ever shown to produce such an outcome (in breast-cancer reduction) it would be worth zillions of dollars as the most impressive drug ever invented in medical history."

Vitamin D levels can be measured in a blood test, and even some of the most conservative doctors are now checking them. While I was undergoing IPT, my vitamin D levels were measured monthly, and if it was not around 50 ng/ml, I was given an injection in my butt to increase it. By the way, these are my favorite supplements to take because they are super small!

DIM

Another powerhouse supplement I take is called DIM. Its full name is Diindolylmethane. DIM is a phytochemical produced during the digestion of cruciferous vegetables such as broccoli, brussel sprouts, cabbage, and cauliflower. DIM is produced from a chemical compound in the vegetables known as indole-3-carbinol or I3C. Research from Memorial Sloan Kettering Cancer Center shows the beneficial effects of DIM on estrogen metabolism, which is the main reason I take six DIM supplements daily. I like taking these; they are small like the vitamin D3.

Curcumin

This natural extract from the spice turmeric should not to be confused with cumin. Turmeric is derived from the plant *Curcuma Longa,* a member of the ginger family. In the lab, curcumin has caused cancer cells to "self-destruct" and can also prevent cancer cells from multiplying. Curcumin has been studied extensively, even by the National Institutes of Health, for its role in preventing and treating cancer. Curcumin may help prevent and treat cancer by several mechanisms. First, it may help block certain dangerous chemicals' cancer-causing effects. It may also block the growth of cancer cells. Additionally, curcumin may stop the growth of blood vessels that are feeding tumors, which in turn prevents the tumors from growing. In the laboratory, curcumin inhibits growth in a large number of cancers, including colon, prostate, lung, liver, stomach, breast, ovarian, and brain cancer, and leukemia. It also forces cancer cells to die. After reading that research I didn't think twice when my two doctors suggested

I take six curcumin supplements daily as well as adding turmeric root to my shake in the morning.

Mushrooms

The last powerhouse supplement I take is a mushroom pill. Mushrooms play an important role in reducing the levels of estrogen in the body and in overall cancer prevention in general. According to Dr. Joel Fuhrman in *Super Immunity*, studies have shown that frequent consumption of mushrooms can decrease the incidence of breast cancer by up to 60 to 70 percent. Similar associations were observed in studies on stomach and colorectal cancers. Dr. Fuhrman goes on to say that the combination of mushrooms and greens is a powerful anticancer cocktail.

"Maitake mushrooms have been shown to have the most pronounced effect on the immune system and are often used in Japan as a complement to chemotherapy to support the immune system," writes Servan-Schreiber in *Anticancer*.

I was hesitant about taking another pill that was yet again a food that I could be adding to my diet. But I admitted to myself that I was having trouble adding mushrooms to my daily diet, so I take two mushroom pills that combine reishi and maitake mushrooms.

Fish Oil/Omega-3s

In addition to the above special anticancer supplements, I take fish oil to help with my intake of omega-3 fatty acids. Research shows that omega-3 fatty acids help protect me from heart disease, stroke, and arthritis as well as overall inflammation in the body that can act as fertilizer for cancer. Omega-3 fatty acids are found in walnuts, flaxseed, and soybeans as well as cold water fish such as trout and salmon. Although I eat walnuts and ground flaxseed every day, I also want the extra protection that the fish oil gives me. It took me awhile to find a brand of fish oil vitamins did not cause me to burp up fish taste, but once I found a brand I liked I had no trouble adding them to my daily handful of vitamins and supplements.

B12

My blood tests indicated that my levels of vitamin B were on the low side, so now I take vitamin B12.

MULTI

The last pill I take is a multivitamin. My doctor helped me choose one that was filled with antioxidants.

TAKEAWAY: MY DAILY SUPPLEMENTS

1. With the help of my doctors I was able to find supplements to help address my estrogen levels.
2. Besides eating my vegetables, I take a broccoli-seed extract supplement.
3. I get my levels of vitamin D3 checked and take a daily supplement.
4. I also add a DIM supplement that helps with the metabolism of estrogen.
5. Curcumin has been shown to stop the growth of blood vessels in tumors, which in turn prevents the tumors from growing.
6. A mushroom pill helps keep my immune system boosted.

TIP 6: MY SUPER-EASY MORNING SHAKE

MY ROCKIN SHAKE

Besides eating my steel-cut oats in the morning, I added a new shake to make my mornings even easier. I was using a combination of separate powders after seeing a lecture by raw food guru David Wolfe. He talks about the importance of adding "superfoods" to your diet. Well, I figured if there was ever a time that I needed more superfoods in my diet, this was it.

David Wolfe describes superfoods as "vibrant, nutritionally dense foods that offer tremendously dietary and healing potential." He explains that plant products such as goji berries, hempseed, cacao beans (raw chocolate), maca, and a host of others represent a uniquely promising piece of the nutritional puzzle. I figured I had nothing to lose by adding some of these superfoods into a morning shake and was adding five or six separate powders and berries. Then at a health expo, I came across a packaged product that included my separate packets in one. Since I would not be putting the separate ingredients into the shake myself, I needed to be sure that the quality of the foods met my standards. I met the owner of Rockin Wellness, Mike Wall. He told me his background story on the product. Wall and his friend Seth started Rockin Wellness because they were looking for a product that contained the best ingredients the world had to offer. Oh, and did I tell you Mike has an adult form of muscular dystrophy and Seth had stage 4 cancer?

The ingredients are all raw (heated to less than 105 degrees and considered "live") and organic. The amazing superfoods in Rockin Wellness are raw organic cacao beans, raw organic goji berries, raw organic hulled hempseeds, organic flaxseed, raw organic maca root, organic green tea, organic yerba mate, raw organic brown rice protein, chia seed, and probiotic—all the things I was trying to get into my diet on a regular basis because of their high nutritional value. I started mixing the shake powder with coconut water (or water); two scoops of Rockin' Wellness; additional ground flax and hulled hempseed, and a handful of walnuts or almonds (all for extra omega-3); and a half cup of frozen wild blueberries (for antioxidants). The shake tastes delicious and is a great way for me to get all these high-quality superfoods in one place. There are three reasons I continue making the shake: I love the way it tastes, it's easy to make, and best of all, and I love how I feel after I drink it! My mornings are my most productive part of the day. I have energy, my mind is clear, and my body is satisfied after drinking the shake. I love this simple addition to my routine to help keep me healthy and build my immunity.

As you can see, I take the food I put into my body pretty seriously. I understand the importance of putting high-quality foods into my body. Are there times when I have a piece of chocolate cake or homemade chocolate chip cookies? Yes there are. My goal is always to do my best when it comes to just about everything, whether it's in regard to food, exercise, or just life in general. I do my best. Do I forget to take my vitamins some days? Yes. Do I have ices in the summertime? Yes. Do you want to know why? Because that's life! Life includes having an Italian ice here and there. Do I indulge often? No, it's all in the big scheme of things. Eating is a social activity. I choose my restaurants carefully. I am lucky enough to have a restaurant close to my home that serves a mostly organic farm-to-table menu. I want to be able to enjoy life and all that it has to offer, and to me that means making smart food choices 90 percent of the time, so I don't feel guilty when I want a taste of something not so healthy. I tune in to how my body feels when I indulge. When I do have a glass of wine, even just a little, I feel the effects. I've found that the "cleaner" I eat, the less I want to indulge. When I do decide to have some dessert, I make sure it is the highest-quality dessert possible and enjoy just a bit. I don't usually eat a whole dessert by myself; I am satisfied with just a couple of bites.

MY LIFE TODAY

I wish I could say having cancer has made me into a wonderful wife, mother, and friend, but it hasn't. I can say it has changed my personality a little. I am less judgmental with myself and with others. I like to think that I have evolved into a calmer person. I am able to feel when things are getting too out of balance in my life. I know when to start saying no to things and how to recognize when too much stress creeps back into my life. I really understand the role of exercise, specifically running and yoga, to help keep me grounded. With the addition of meditation every day, I am able to focus on the here and now. I think of my diet as an upgraded version of an already pretty healthy diet. I now drink green shakes daily—something I would never have even considered before.

A friend recently told me that her cancer was in remission. It made me think, *Is that how I'm supposed to think about my cancer?* It's funny, but I have always thought of myself as cancer-free. The word *remission* sounds like the cancer cells are still there just sleeping. I want to think of myself as not having this disease anymore. I don't even know if the word *remission* relates to breast cancer, but I don't like it, so I'm not using it.

I leave you with one last song.

> Steve Winwood's "Higher Love"
> Think about it   there must be a higher love,
> Down in the heart or hidden in the stars above
> Without it time is wasted time
> Look inside your heart, I'll look inside mine

Recipes

WELCOME TO MY GO-TO, SUPER-EASY, super-doable recipes. I use these recipes to get all my healthy antioxidants into my diet without even realizing they are there. I like to experiment with cooking and am always trying new recipes or thinking of ways to add more good stuff to each meal. I have two very special friends who helped me develop many of these recipes.

Tina Annibell is my health coach friend who is an awesome cook and loves teaching others how to incorporate healthy habits into their busy lives. Visit her at www.nourishedliving.net.

Linda Davis is a stage 4 ovarian cancer survivor and cancer health coach. She teaches people how to incorporate juicing and blending fruits and vegetables into their daily routine. Visit her at www.vegoutwithlinda.com.

Thank you both for your friendship and sharing your knowledge. You inspire me to keep cooking and using foods to help myself heal.

I am constantly reminding myself that cooking is meant to be simple. Nothing fancy needs to be done to the food when you use fresh, organic, high-quality ingredients. If the recipe calls for meat, be sure it is organic free-range. I now treat meat as a condiment. What I mean is that just a little bit of meat goes a long way toward adding flavor to a soup or stew. I rarely eat just a plain piece of meat.

I remind myself all the time to have fun cooking and preparing food, because all that energy is going into the food itself. I put on music, ask the kids to help, relax, and know that preparing my own food is a huge gift in today's world. And most important, I remind myself that the food I put into my body is just as powerful as any medicine.

Breakfast Ideas

Steel-Cut Oats

One of the first upgrades to a higher-nutrient diet started with steel-cut oats. I learned that not all oatmeal is created equal. Some kinds have more nutritional value than others. Most oats are refined, but I always look for steel-cut oats. *Steel cut* means just that: the oat is cut into two or three pieces by a steel blade. Steel-cut oats take longer to digest than refined (rolled oats), helps me stay fuller longer, and has a stabilizing effect on my insulin levels (no sugar highs or lows).

> 4 Servings
> 1 cup steel-cut oats
> 3 cups water

1. Bring water to a boil.
2. Add oats.
3. Cook covered for 10–20 minutes (depending how chewy you like the cereal).
4. Stir occasionally (so the cereal doesn't stick to the bottom of the pot).
5. Remove when consistency is good and let stand for 2–3 minutes.

These oats make the perfect base to which you can add more healthy foods such as fresh or frozen fruit, ground flaxseed, chopped nuts (walnuts, raw almonds), or cinnamon. This is one of my favorite dishes year-round.

Rockin' Wellness Smoothie

When I am pressed for time in the morning and want a high-quality, super-packed smoothie, I turn to my friends at Rockin Wellness. This product has all the ingredients I was putting in separately. The flavor of the Rockin Wellness powder is so good that I can add lots of high-nutrient extras without sacrificing taste. Remember, if the smoothie doesn't taste good, I won't drink it.

> 2 scoops Rockin Wellness
> 12 ounces coconut water (or plain water)

½ frozen banana
½ cup frozen or fresh blueberries
1 tablespoon "greens" powder
¼ cup of ground flaxseed
¼ cup of hempseed
Handful of walnuts or almonds

Blend and enjoy!

Bonus: Add a handful of organic spinach or a handful of organic kale to make it SUPER!

SUPERFOOD CEREAL

(Contributed by Suzanne Boothby: www.suzanneboothby.com)

1 apple, chopped
1 handful of goji berries
1 handful of seeds: try sunflower, pumpkin, hemp, or a mix
1 handful of nuts: try walnuts, almonds, cashews, pecans or a mix
½ handful of cacao nibs
1 sprinkle of coconut flakes
1 sprinkle of ground flaxseeds

Put all ingredients in a bowl and then pour in your favorite milk (try almond, hemp, or coconut).

Energizing Buckwheat Pancakes

(Contributed by Suzanne Boothby: www.suzanneboothby.com)

Makes about 8 medium-size pancakes.

> ½ cup buckwheat flour
> 1 egg
> 1 cup almond milk
> 1 tablespoon maple syrup
> Sea salt to taste
> Butter

Add buckwheat flour to a large mixing bowl with a little sea salt to taste. In a separate bowl crack the egg, and add the milk and the maple syrup. Then pour the liquid mixture into the flour mixture and stir until all ingredients are combined. Mixture should be light and flow easily off a spoon. Heat a flat pancake pan with a dab of butter. Use a measuring cup to pour your mixture. Flip when you see bubbles start to form throughout. Top with blueberries and maple syrup.

Smoothies and Juices

One of the biggest changes since my diagnosis of cancer has been the addition of smoothies and juices. The easiest way to distinguish between a smoothie and a juice is that one is made in a blender and the other is made with a juicer. Remember to take it slow and add more fruit if necessary. There is no exact science to smoothie or juice making; mine are rarely the exact same. As I experiment, I write down what I liked about the drink and what I didn't so I can replicate it again (or not). I love adding a frozen banana to my smoothie—it makes it cold as well as creamy. Another tip is to put the drink into a special glass. I like to use a goblet or special glass jar with my glass straw.

I Love Me Smoothie

> 1 ripe frozen banana
> 1 ripe pear or 1 red apple, sliced
> 1½ cups almond milk, coconut water, or plain water
> 2 heaping tablespoons almond butter or cashew butter
> 1 very large kale leaf or 2 medium kale leaves (center stems removed)
> 4 ice cubes

Place all ingredients in a blender, blend until smooth. Enjoy!

Bonus: Add 1 tablespoon chia seeds. Chia seeds are an excellent source of fiber, packed with antioxidants, full of protein, and loaded with vitamins and minerals, and are the richest known plant source of omega-3.

Berry Smoothie + a Touch of Green

> 1/2 cup raw organic cashews (soaked) or 2 tablespoons nut
> butter (cashew or almond)
> 1/2 cup almond milk or coconut milk
> 1 tablespoon chia seeds
> 2 large handfuls baby spinach
> 1/4 cup frozen raspberries
> 1/4 cup fresh or frozen blueberries or blackberries
> 1/2 frozen banana

Put the soaked nuts and milk in a blender. Puree until smooth. Add remaining ingredients and puree until smooth. If you have a high-power blender, skip the brief soaking and blend everything.

Note: If you want to try raw organic nuts such as cashews, try soaking them for about 1–3 hours to get them softer. If soaking the nuts isn't an option, try experimenting with various nut butters like almond or cashew.

Other things to add to smoothies: Add some hempseeds, which have a near perfect ratio of omega-3-6-9, or some ground flaxseeds. Flaxseeds are rich in omega-3 fatty acids, which help fight inflammation in the body and are high in fiber. Flaxseeds are perhaps our best source of lignans, which convert in our intestines to substances that tend to balance female hormones. There is evidence that lignans may promote fertility, reduce perimenopausal symptoms, and help prevent breast cancer. Both hempseeds and ground flaxseeds are great ways to add protein and cancer-fighting properties to your diet without noticing the taste.

Orange Galore Juice

> 2 organic juice oranges (peeled)
> 4 organic carrots
> 1 small knob ginger
> High-quality ground cinnamon, to taste

Put oranges, carrots, and ginger through a juicer. Sprinkle with cinnamon, stir, and enjoy!

GREEN GIANT JUICE

     2–3 leaves of organic Lacinato kale

     1 lemon, washed, with ends trimmed off

     1 large organic cucumber

     3–4 stalks of celery, including the leafy top

     1–2 organic green apples

Juice the above and finish with an extra squeeze of lemon and/or lime.

Soups

Soups make a perfect meal in all seasons. They are great in the winter when all that's available are root vegetables and perfect in the summer when there are lots of greens around to pump up the nutritional value of your meal. Soups are easy to make, can be eaten for several meals, and are usually even tastier the next day. When using canned beans, be sure the cans are BPA-free and the beans don't contain extra salt or preservatives. Look for beans that have been cooked with kombu (seaweed), which aids in digestion. Another tip is to rinse the beans in a colander, ridding them of phytic acid, which is what causes gas.

White Bean and Green Soup

This recipe was adapted from Ina Garten's *The Barefoot Contessa Cookbook*. It has long been a staple in my house in the summer. This soup is also great the next day. Sometimes I even add another can of cannellini beans to the leftover soup to get another meal.

Serves 4

> 2 tablespoons extra virgin olive oil or coconut oil
> 1 garlic clove, minced
> 1 large yellow onion
> 2 BPA-free cans of white cannellini beans
> 1 quart vegetable stock
> 1 branch fresh rosemary, 3–4 inches (or 1 tablespoon dried)
> 1 bay leaf
> Kosher Salt and freshly ground black pepper to taste

In a large stockpot over medium heat, add olive oil or coconut oil. Add onions and cook until translucent (about 5 minutes). Add garlic and sauté for another 2 minutes. Add rinsed beans, vegetable stock, and bay leaf, rosemary branch, salt and pepper, and bring to a boil over high heat. Simmer for 30 minutes. Remove bay leaf and rosemary branch. Take about half the soup and put it in a blender (or use an immersion blender) and blend until creamy. Return soup to pot and stir.

Bonus: Add handfuls of roughly chopped kale (or any other hearty green) and simmer for another 20 minutes.

Black Bean Soup

This is a simple 10-minute go-to soup that can be blended, left thick and chunky, or be served somewhere in between.

(Contributed by Tina Annibell, www.nourishedliving.net)

Serves 4

> 2 tablespoons extra virgin olive oil or coconut oil
> 4 cloves of garlic, minced
> 1 teaspoon cumin (plus a pinch more)
> 1 cup organic salsa (any brand and "heat")
> 2 15-ounce BPA-free cans of black beans, rinsed and drained
> 1 cup homemade vegetable stock, store-bought organic vegetable stock, or water

Rinse beans until the foam is gone. In a saucepan over medium heat, sauté garlic and cumin in olive oil for 3 minutes. Add salsa and cook for 1–2 minutes. Add beans and broth, and stir. Let simmer 5 minutes. Remove half the soup and put in a blender on low. Return to the pot and stir. Optional: Top with green onions.

Bonus: Add shredded greens (try kale, collards, or spinach) to soup pot and simmer for another 20 minutes.

LEMONY LENTIL SOUP WITH LEEKS

From a health perspective, lentils help stimulate cancer-preventing enzymes and help lower estrogen levels in the body. Women who eat lentils (and beans in general) have a lower risk of developing breast cancer thanks to their antioxidants and fiber, according to the *International Journal of Cancer*.

(Contributed by Suzanne Boothby, www.suzanneboothby.com)

Serves 4

> 1 tablespoon butter (or use a little bit of water for a vegan version)
> 2 leeks, green and white parts, sliced into half moons
> 3 large carrots, diced
> 1 cup lentils
> 1 lemon, juiced
> 1 bunch parsley, chopped
> 4 kale leaves, chopped
> Salt and pepper to taste
> 2–3 cups water (you can make this soup thicker or more watery, depending on how much you use)

Heat the butter in a soup pot over medium heat. Add the leeks and carrots and cook for about 3 minutes. Add the lentils and stir for a few moments, and then add the water. Let the mixture cook with the top on for about 10 minutes or so. Add the lemon juice, parsley and kale, and cook for another 5–7 minutes. Add salt and pepper to taste. When the lentils are soft, this soup is ready to eat.

Irish Potato and Cabbage Soup

This is one of those recipes where meat is added as a condiment. The simplicity of the ingredients makes this soup perfect in the winter when the local food includes root vegetables.

(Contributed by Tina Annibell, www.nourishedliving.net)

Serves 6–8

> 3 tablespoons olive oil
> 1 large white onion, diced
> 4 garlic cloves, minced
> Small head of cabbage, cored and sliced thinly (about 6 cups)
> 4 medium gold or white potatoes, peeled and cut into cubes
> 2 large carrots, peeled and diced
> 4 sausages (you can omit if you want to make it meatless)
> 6–8 cups organic vegetable broth
> Sea salt and pepper to taste
> 1 Tbsp apple cider vinegar

Heat olive oil in a large soup pot over medium heat. Add the onion and a pinch of sea salt, and cook for about 5 minutes. Add garlic and cabbage and stir together; cook until the cabbage has wilted. Add potatoes, carrots, and sausages. Stir. Add between 6-8 cups organic vegetable broth. Season with salt and pepper. Cover and bring to a high simmer, then lower the heat and simmer until the vegetables are fork tender, about 45 minutes. Right before you are ready to serve, splash a touch of apple cider vinegar on it to liven things up.

SQUASH AND WHITE BEAN SOUP

(Contributed by Peggy Buresh, www.PeggyLivingWell.com)

Serves 4

> 1 tablespoon olive oil
> 1 onion, chopped
> 1 14.5-ounce can chopped tomatoes
> 1 small butternut squash, peeled and cubed into ½" pieces
> 1 tablespoon dried thyme
> 5 cups of water or vegetable broth
> 2 15-ounce cans cannellini beans, rinsed
> 1 bunch chopped spinach or kale
> sea salt and black pepper to taste

In soup pot, heat oil, add onion, and cook until the onion is soft (about 5–6 minutes). Add tomatoes, with juice included. Cook for another 3 minutes or more. Stir in the squash, thyme, 5 cups of water or broth, and salt and pepper, and bring to a boil. Reduce heat and simmer until squash is tender (about 15–20 minutes. Stir in the beans and spinach, and cook till the spinach is wilted and the beans are heated through (about 2–3 minutes). Serve with your favorite hearty bread.

STEWS

I really enjoy stews because they are so simple. You can easily double the recipe to get enough to serve as lunch the next day, and it's a great way to get in those healthy beans.

LENTIL STEW

Serves 4

This recipe is simple and takes a little more than 30 minutes from start to finish. It calls for burdock root, which is long like a carrot with dark brown skin that looks like dirt. (You don't need to scrub that away—just give it a good wash.) It is very fibrous, and people say it tastes like artichoke. Known for its medicinal properties, it should be available at your local health food store. The recipe also includes Umeboshi plum vinegar, which is also known for its medicinal properties. It is a great digestive aid with a salty taste that is perfect for drizzling on soups and stews.

> 1 tablespoon olive oil (or coconut oil)
> 1 teaspoon of ground cumin
> 1 large onion, diced
> 2 large carrots cut into half moons
> 2 burdock roots (optional) cut into small, thin half moons
> 2 cups dried red lentils
> 6 cups of water
> 1 teaspoon umeboshi plum vinegar

Heat oil in a pot over medium heat. Add cumin and cook, stirring, for about 30 seconds. Add onions and cook 5 minutes. Add carrot and burdock root, and sauté another 3 minutes. Add lentils and water and cook for about 20–30 minutes, until lentils and roots are soft. Before serving, splash umeboshi vinegar, stir and enjoy.

Bonus: Add a handful of kale cut into small pieces and simmer in soup for 15–20 minutes before serving.

Black Bean and Sweet Potato Stew

This dish can be made either in a large pot or in a slow cooker. When I use canned beans, I thoroughly rinse them in a colander to remove some of their gas-producing properties. This stew can be eaten alone or over brown rice, or try the ancient grain quinoa. Quinoa has been grown and consumed for more than 8,000 years and is grown in the Andes Mountains. Quinoa is a high-protein grain with B vitamins, iron, zinc, potassium, calcium, and vitamin E.

Serves 4

> 1 medium onion, chopped
> 2 cans black beans
> 3 medium sweet potatoes, peeled and diced into 2-inch pieces
> 1 small can (or glass) organic tomato paste
> 32 ounces vegetable broth (either makes your own or looks for an organic brand)
> 2 teaspoons each: salt, pepper, cumin, coriander
> 1 dried bay leaf

Put chopped onions, diced sweet potatoes, and black beans into slow cooker (or large pot). Pour vegetable broth over the above foods and stir. You may need to adjust the liquid; add some water if it looks low. Add bay leaf, cumin, and coriander. Cook on low 6–8 hours or until sweet potatoes are fork tender. If you are using a large pot, simmer for about 40–60 minutes until sweet potatoes are fork tender. When the potatoes are done, add the tomato paste, salt, and pepper, and remove the bay leaf. This can be eaten alone or over brown rice or experiment with quinoa.

Easy Stewing Vegetables

(Contributed by Rochelle Blank-Zimmer, www.yournaturalchoice.net)

Serves 4

1 medium onion, chopped
1–2 cloves garlic, chopped
Handful of mushrooms, chopped (or any mixed veggies you
  like)
½ head cauliflower, chopped
1 cup peas
1 carrot, chopped
1 zucchini, chopped
½ red pepper, chopped
1 28-ounce container of chunky tomatoes or fresh

Wild or brown rice
Cumin
Turmeric
Coriander
Garlic powder
Tiny amount of fresh ginger
Salt/pepper to taste, optional

Cook rice. In a soup pot, add onions and steam-sauté for a few minutes, stirring constantly and adding a tablespoon or two of water as needed. Add garlic. Add mushrooms and cauliflower, and continue steam-sautéing, stirring occasionally. Add peas, carrots, zucchini, red pepper, and tomatoes.

Add small amounts of cumin, turmeric, coriander, salt/pepper, garlic powder, and fresh ginger.

First bring to boil, then simmer, stirring occasionally, for about 10–15 minutes.

Tips for Prepping Greens

How to clean greens

When you purchase green lettuces from a local farmer, farm stand, or farmers' market, it is usually coming straight from the earth, so it is important to get all that dirt off the leaves before eating. It's no fun making a beautiful salad only to bite into a grain of sand. The perfect way to easily clean your greens is with a salad spinner.

One tip I learned from Chef Peter Berley is to really dry your greens. "If your greens aren't thoroughly dry, the dressing won't cling to them and your salad will be soggy and tasteless," he says. "Avoid this by firing up your salad spinner not once, but twice: spin the greens dry, pour the water out of the spinner bowl, shake the greens to wake them from their spun torpor, and then spin them again—you'll be amazed by how much more water you will get the second time around."

Another tip: When washing your greens in the salad spinner, fill the container only halfway. Resist the urge to fill it completely; this way each leaf has the opportunity to get completely clean.

How to make your own salad dressing

When I make my own salads, 99 percent of the time I make my own dressings too. One reason is that it is so simple to make homemade dressing. Another is that I can control the ingredients. I know which type of oil I used (because I want to avoid vegetable, corn, soy, canola, and safflower oils) and that there are no hidden ingredients that I don't want, such as MSG or sugar.

Vinaigrette in a Jar

(From Maggie at the Golden Earthworm Farm in Jamesport, Long Island, who adapted it from Jacques Pepin)

> 2 teaspoons chopped garlic
> 2 tablespoons Dijon-style mustard
> 1/2 teaspoon kosher salt
> 1/4 teaspoon freshly ground black pepper
> 1/4 cup red- or white-wine vinegar
> 1 cup extra-virgin olive oil

Put all the ingredients in a jar, screw on the lid, and shake very well. Taste and adjust the seasonings, adding more oil or vinegar as you like. Store in the refrigerator up to 2 weeks, and shake to blend before using.

How to properly dress your greens

Now that you have cleaned and dried your fresh lettuce and made the perfect salad dressing, you want to be sure you use the perfect amount. A tip I learned from Chef Peter Berley is to put the clean, dry lettuce leaves in a large bowl, pour the dressing around the perimeter of the bowl, and use your hands to mix the lettuce and dressing together. When you pour the dressing around the sides of the bowl and not over the center of the salad you tend to use the perfect amount of dressing. Every time I use this tip, the salad-to-dressing ratio is perfect.

How to sauté greens

My introduction to sautéed greens was with a big leafy green vegetable called Swiss chard. I had never tasted it until it was in my CSA farm share. I read the farm's newsletter to learn how to cook it. The recipe was so simple that it became the base for all my greens.

This recipe is adapted from Cait Johnson.

> 1 bunch Swiss chard
> 1 tablespoon olive oil (or coconut oil)

1 tablespoon chopped fresh rosemary
1/3 cup dark raisins or golden raisins
2 tablespoons pine nuts
Salt and freshly ground black pepper, to taste

Remove the chard stems and the thick central vein from each leaf. Chop the leaves very coarsely. Using a large, heavy-bottomed frying pan over medium high heat, add oil. Add the chard and the rosemary, stirring well to coat the chard with the oil mixture. Cook, stirring constantly, for another minute until the chard has wilted to about half its original volume. Add raisins and pine nuts, stirring to combine evenly, and continue cooking until any moisture has evaporated. The entire cooking process should take no more than about 3 minutes. Season with salt and pepper and serve immediately.

How to store your greens

According to my farmer (the Golden Earthworm), the best way for me to store my green lettuces is in perforated plastic bags wrapped in a damp paper towel and then kept in the refrigerator vegetable crisper. I usually use a Green Bag from Debbie Meyer. The bags are made of a natural mineral (BPA-free) that helps extends the life and freshness of fruits and vegetables. When I receive my vegetables from the farm, I quickly rinse them off, dry them, put them in the bags, and then refrigerate.

Tips on making greens taste great

My two tips for making sautéed greens taste great are to add two simple ingredients. The first is sea salt. Sea salt is different from table salt. Table salt is highly refined, all the trace minerals are removed, and a bleaching agent is added to create the pure white color. In contrast, sea salt is sun dried and contains a high mineral content. The best part about using a high-quality sea salt is that a little goes a long way. I like to use Himalayan or Celtic sea salts. I add it to sautéed greens at the very end and remember to use just a pinch.

My other tip on making greens taste great is to include a squeeze of lemon. Just a little lemon juice helps take away any of the bitterness the greens may have. When I'm finished squeezing the lemon, I place the lemon wedge on the plate, and the yellow contrast with the greens make it not only taste great, but look good too.

Spinach Salad with Citrus Vinaigrette

1 package baby spinach (about 7 ounces)
½ cup feta cheese
¼ small red onion, very thinly sliced
1/3 cup sliced almonds
1 orange, peeled, seeded, and cut into ½-inch chunks

Dressing
1/3 cup extra virgin olive oil
1/3 cup fresh squeezed orange juice (1 Valencia orange)
1/8 cup white balsamic vinegar
1 tablespoon Dijon mustard
Sea salt and pepper to taste

Make dressing in medium-size bowl. Then add the feta cheese, onions, almonds, and oranges together. Be sure everything is coated with dressing. Put the spinach into a big bowl and toss with the dressing, cheese, onions, almonds, and oranges.

SNACKS

I am always looking for healthy snacks for my family and me. Having healthy snacks on hand helps us fuel our bodies well and not give in to tempting junk foods when we are having an energy crash.

NUTS AND SEEDS

My go-to snack is usually a handful of raw organic nuts or seeds such as walnuts, almonds, sunflower seeds, and pumpkin seeds. Our new favorite is tamari almonds. Nuts and seeds are simple to eat and contain all those healthy antioxidants.

FRUIT AND NUT BUTTER

Another favorite snack is a piece of fruit (I love to use apples or pears) cut into pieces. Then I dip the fruit into a raw nut butter like almond butter or cashew butter. I prefer the taste of almond or cashew butter over regular peanut butter. I go to Whole Foods and grind my own nut butters at their bulk station so I am sure no other ingredients were added.

FROZEN BANANA DESSERT

As a special dessert treat I love putting a frozen banana in the blender or food processor and then adding raw cacao chips, shredded coconut, and a handful of chopped nuts. It has become my version of Chunky Monkey.

VEGETABLES AND HUMMUS

Hummus is a mixture of ground chickpeas, garlic, and usually tahini (ground sesame seeds). It is quite easy to make in a blender, but I admit sometimes I cheat and purchase hummus from the store. I cut vegetables from the garden like carrots, radish, and broccoli and put hummus out on a tray. People don't even realize they are eating a bean dip.

This recipe is adapted from Ina Garten.

1 16-ounce BPA-free can of chickpeas (also called garbanzo beans)

¼ cup of the liquid from the can of chickpeas
Juice of ½ lemon
1½ tablespoons of tahini (crushed sesame seeds)
2 cloves garlic, crushed
½ teaspoon salt
2 tablespoons or more of extra virgin olive oil

Drain chickpeas and set aside ¼ cup liquid. Combine remaining ingredients in blender or food processor. Add the ¼ cup chickpea liquid and blend for 3–5 minutes. For a creamier texture add more olive oil.

KALE CHIPS

When my then ten-year-old ate these up, I knew I had a hit on my hands. They are simple to make and take only a few ingredients.

1 bunch of Lacinato kale (a.k.a. dinosaur kale—because the
kale looks like dinosaur skin)
Sea salt
Extra virgin olive oil (or coconut oil)

Preheat oven to 425 degrees. Rinse kale and remove the stems. This can be done by holding a kale leaf by the stem and with one hand using the thumb and index finger on your other hand to pull in a downward motion. Pour olive oil into a small bowl, and with your fingers, lightly coat the kale with the olive oil.

Lay the kale on a cookie sheet lined with parchment paper. Sprinkle lightly with sea salt. Cook for approximately 5–6 minutes, depending on your oven. You want the kale to be a little brown, and the chips should be mostly green with brown patches. They will burn quickly, so keep an eye on them. Let them cool and enjoy.

MEALS

TURKEY AND BEAN CHILI

    1 tablespoon extra virgin olive oil
    1 onion, chopped
    1 jalapeno pepper, diced
    4 cloves of garlic, minced
    2 red bell peppers, chopped
    1 pound ground turkey
    2 teaspoons ground cumin
    1 tablespoon chili powder
    1 15-ounce can pinto beans
    1 15-ounce can black beans
    1 28-ounce can diced tomatoes
    1½ cups chicken broth
    Sea salt and pepper to taste

Heat oil in large pot over medium heat. Add onions and jalapeno and cook for 3 minutes. Stir in garlic and peppers and cook for 4 minutes or until peppers start to become tender. Stir in turkey, break up with a fork, and cook another 5 minutes or until the turkey is browned. Stir in cumin and chili powder. Add beans, tomatoes, broth, salt and pepper. Bring heat to high and allow to boil. Reduce heat and simmer for 5–10 minutes.

Bonus: Serve over brown rice or quinoa for a really satisfying meal.

VEGETABLES AND PASTA

My ultimate go-to dish is my vegetable and pasta dish. I make this when I have vegetables on hand and they need to be used up. I experiment with different types of pasta. Sometimes I use fresh pasta from my local Italian market, quinoa pasta, rice pasta, wheat pasta, or even a butternut-squash frozen ravioli. The key to adding the vegetables is to be sure they are cut into small, bite-size pieces. I top off the dish with either pesto or organic tomato red sauce. Here is a sample of one I threw together the other night.

> 1 package of quinoa pasta
> 1 tablespoon extra-virgin olive oil or coconut oil
> 1 small onion cut in strips
> 1 handful of fresh green beans cut in half
> 2 carrots in long strips
> 1 zucchini, cut in half and then into half-moon shape
> 2 pieces of Lacinato kale, roughly chopped minus the stem
> 3 handfuls of spinach, roughly chopped

In a large stockpot, boil water for pasta. In a large sauté pan, heat oil and add onion. Next add the vegetables that cook the longest, green beans, then carrots, zucchini, kale, and then spinach. I add some pasta water to the vegetables to add some liquid. When the pasta is done, strain it, add it to the sauté pan, and stir everything together. Add any sauce at this point (try pesto, tomato, or olive oil). Put in a big bowl and top with basil.

Pesto Sauce

> 2 cloves garlic
> ½ cup olive oil
> ¼ cup pignoli or pumpkin seeds
> Sea salt to taste
> 2 cups any greens (either traditional basil, or try arugula, spinach, or kale)
> Optional: ¼ cup locatelli Romano or parmesan cheese

In a food processor, blend together garlic, olive oil, nuts, and sea salt. Add greens and process to a very finely chopped, paste consistency.

Note: Pesto freezes well. Add a dollop to white bean soup, lentil soup, pasta dishes, or hummus.

Bonus Guide

PRODUCTS

All-Clad is the cookware I switched to after my cancer journey. All-Clad is an American company that uses stainless steel to produce a complete line of superior cookware. www.all-clad.com

Deodorant: I switched to a chemical-free deodorant called Pit Putty that is made by an online company called Bumble and Bee. I have been through many deodorants, and this product seems to work. Bumble and Bee are so sure your body will respond to one of their scents that they offer a special replacement guarantee.

Dr. Bronner's Magic Soaps are amazingly versatile. They are castile soaps, which means they are completely vegetable-oil based with no animal products. All the soaps are USDA-certified organic and 100 percent biodegradable. I use it in the shower, as well as to clean the kitchen countertop and floors. I even do laundry with it. Soaps come in peppermint, lavender, almond, tea tree, eucalyptus, rose, and citrus orange natural scents. www.drbronners.com

Environmental Working Group is the nation's leading environmental health research and advocacy organization. Their mission is to serve as a watchdog to see that Americans get straight facts, unfiltered and unspun, so they can make healthier choices and enjoy a cleaner environment. www. ewg.org

Fat, Sick & Nearly Dead is a documentary that follows the sixty-day journey of Australian Joe Cross, who traveled across the United States while juice fasting to regain his health under the care of Dr. Joel Fuhrman. www.fatsickandnearlydead.com

Food Matters is a documentary about nutrition, exploring malnutrition and causes of cancer. www.FoodMatters.com

Fresh the Movie is a film that tells the stories of "real people" rediscovering "real food." *Fresh* represents a powerful way for you to educate yourself and your community on living a healthy, local, and sustainable life through food. www.freshthemovie.com

Hungry for Change is another food documentary that guides you toward making healthier food choices. www.Hungryforchange.com

Insulin Potentiation Therapy is an alternative cancer treatment using insulin to administer low-dose chemotherapy. www.LinchitzWellness.com

IV Vitamin C Therapy was part of my cancer treatment therapy. Vitamin C in IV form is shown to enhance the immune system.

John Masters Organics Products is a line of hair care, skin care, and body care products. All the ingredients are organic, and do not contain sodium lauryl sulfate, parabens, artificial colors, fragrance, or fillers. I use the shampoo, conditioner, facial creams, and body wash. www.JohnMasters.com

Livestrong: The Lance Armstrong Foundation unites, inspires, and empowers those affected by cancer. The Fertile Hope program is dedicated to providing reproductive information, support, and hope to cancer patients and survivors whose medical treatments present the risk of infertility. www.livestrong.org

May I Be Frank is a documentary that follows the transformation of Frank Ferrante's life. Frank turns his life over for forty-two days to three guys who coach him physically, emotionally, and spiritually. He eats only raw food, practices gratitude, and visits local holistic practitioners. This is one of my favorite inspirational movies. Frank lets us into his life in a very real way. www.MayIBeFrankmovie.com

Meditation: I turn to one from my favorite authors and speaker, Deepak Chopra. He offers free twenty-one-day meditations throughout the year. www.chopracentermeditation.com

Melaleuca is a company that offers a complete line of nontoxic products for the home. I used the *Renew* body lotion on my radiated breast to keep the skin from scarring. www.melaleuca.com

Oncotype DX is a diagnostic test that quantifies the likelihood of disease recurrence in women with early stage breast cancer.

Omega Juicer 8006 is a masticating-style juicer. The dual-stage juice processing system extracts the maximum amount of juice from fruits, vegetables, and leafy greens. I bought it because it was in my price range (around $300) and was easy to clean. I am very happy with it.

Rockin Wellness is an organic and raw powdered drink mix. The ingredients in RW are all things that I used separately that are now in one package: cacao, goji berry, maca, hempseed, flaxseed, green tea, yerba mate, and more. I love the taste and mix it with greens, half a frozen banana, and frozen blueberries as my morning shake. www.rockinwellness.com

TED Talks is a program of a nonprofit, TED, devoted to ideas worth spreading. It started out in 1984 as a conference bringing together people from three worlds: technology, entertainment, and design. www.ted.com

Vitamix is much more than a blender; it is in a class of its own. The Vitamix allows you to chop, blend, cream, puree, and more. This is the only machine I use to make my daily smoothie; it pulverizes kale, spinach, and ice in seconds. www.vitamix.com

Vitacost is an online retailer and direct marketer of health and wellness products, including dietary supplements such as vitamins, cosmetics, food, and personal care products all at discounted rates. www.Vitacost.com

Young Living Oils, Lavender Essential Oil. Young Living Essential Oils is the world leader in the production of pure, food-grade essential oils. I used the lavender oil on my lumpectomy scar and on my radiated breast tissue. www.YoungLiving.com

PEOPLE

Shawn Anchor is the author of the international best seller *The Happiness Advantage.* Shawn is regarded as one of the world's leading experts on the connection between happiness and success. www.ShawnAnchor.com

Tina Annibell is a holistic nutrition counselor and offers nutrition coaching, cooking instruction, and organic gardening classes on Long Island, New York. www.NourishedLiving.net

Peter Berley is a chef, cookbook author, and culinary instructor. Peter's foremost concern is the development of local sustainable food systems and the fate of home cooking in America. www.PeterBerley.com

Dr. William Bezmen, PhD, RN, and co-director of Pathways to Health, has been working with people to develop their inner senses for self-empowerment and healing for more than thirty years. www. pathwaystohealth.com

Suzanne Boothby is author of *The After Cancer Diet: How to Live Healthier Than Ever Before.* This book empowers cancer thrivers to improve their health through simple and sustainable diet and lifestyle changes. www. suzanneboothby.com

Peggy Buresh is an RN and health coach specializing in hormonal imbalances and weight loss. www.PeggyLivingWell.com

Maureen Calamia is a feng shui consultant on Long Island. Maureen helps people create a home and business that bring joy and harmony into their lives, with site orientation and geographical analysis, the artful placement of furniture and objects, and incorporation of harmony, balance, and natural elements. www.luminous-spaces.com

Kris Carr is the person behind the Crazy, Sexy, Cancer brand. She made a documentary with that name and has released many best-selling books. Kris is a cancer thriver, best-selling author, speaker, and wellness coach. www.KrisCarr.com

Linda Davis is a certified health coach who works with people and families who are affected by cancer. www.Veg-outwithlinda.com

Dr. Joel Fuhrman is an MD and best-selling author who specializes in treating ailments with nutrition. My favorite of his books is *Super Immunity.* www.drfuhrman.com

Bonnie Gayle is the maker of Sex Butter personal lubricant. Sex Butter is made of organic essential oils, and it's paraben- and hormone-free. www. sexbutter.net

Glamorganic Goddess is a blog and website that reviews natural, organic beauty products written by breast cancer thriver Danielle Messina. www. glamorganicgoddess.com

Dr. Mark Hyman is an MD and author. He has dedicated his career to identifying and addressing the root cause of chronic illness through the practice of functional medicine, which addresses the underlying causes of disease engaging both patient and practitioner. His practice is in Lenox, Massachusetts. My favorite book of his is *UltraMetabolism.* www.drhyman. com

Joyce and Kevin O'Brien. Within a five-year period, Joyce O'Brien's husband, Kevin, was paralyzed after a brain hemorrhage, and both Joyce and Kevin received diagnoses of late-stage cancers. Joyce's life mission was to research and study with top doctors and experts in the holistic health field to discover what makes us sick and how to heal. Joyce is the author of *Choose to Live* and *Being Cancer Free*. www.joyceobrien.com

Lorraine Miller is the author of *From Gratitude to Bliss*. This book offers a step-by-step guide to incorporating daily gratitude into your life. www.NourishbyNature.com

Barbara Musser is the author of *Sexy After Cancer*. She is a breast cancer survivor and motivational speaker; she helps post cancer women get in touch with their inner Aphrodite. www.SexyAfterCancer.com

Michael Pollan is an author, journalist, and food activist. My favorite of his books is *Food Rules*. www.MichaelPollan.com

Tony Robbins is a self-help author and motivational speaker. www.TonyRobbins.com

David Servan-Schrieber is the author of *Anticancer: A New Way of Life*. His book is part memoir of his own journey with brain cancer and part textbook with information on cancer cells and how they work. The book draws on both conventional and alternative ways to slow and prevent cancer.

Tamara St. John is a breast cancer thriver who is a wealth of information when it comes to alternative health solutions. www.TamaraStJohn.com. Her book is called *Defeat Cancer Now*.

Rochelle Blank Zimmer is a holistic health coach and educator specializing in conscious eating with plant-based nutrition. www.YourNaturalChoice.net

PLACES

Dr. Linchitz Medical Wellness: The mission of this medical practice based on Long Island, New York, is to help patients achieve vibrant health by emphasizing natural treatment and preventing illness. www.linchitzwellness.com

Institute of Integrative Nutrition: The world's largest nutrition school and my alma mater. www.integrativenutrition.com

About the Author

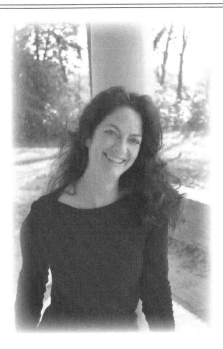

After graduating college, Christine Egan started her career as an account supervisor for an advertising agency, working on a major fast food account. She left her corporate life to be a wife and mom. She pursued her passion for health and nutrition by attending The New York School for Massage Therapy and The Institute for Integrative Nutrition. While starting a private nutrition practice and serving as the director of a local food movement organization; she discovered she had cancer. Determined to stay healthy, Christine blogged about her cancer journey and ran a half marathon just after completing radiation. She now lives with her husband, their three kids, and Zoe the dog in Bayport, New York.

CPSIA information can be obtained at www.ICGtesting.com
Printed in the USA
LVOW01s1440031013

355310LV00017B/708/P